"Understanding healing at its many levels, the physical, psychological, spiritual, and experiential, is Noah's life's work. With this book, he hopes to coax and challenge caregivers to take a deeper look into their own lives and practice styles so that they may more readily create an extraordinary healing environment and presence that prompts and supports their patients' transition to better health."

—*M. Chris Link, M.D., Integrative Medicine*
Practitioner, Jefferson City, MO

"Noah asks the question, 'Can we make the client feel safe?' The creation of the therapeutic space is perhaps one of the greatest skills necessary in the bodyworker's repertoire but, bizarrely, it is also one so very rarely taught. This text is dense with information but written with accessibility in mind—mirroring Noah's own approach to his therapy—approachable, supportive and clear, but with a depth of understanding at its core. It will open the door to many explorations and give the mindful therapist the necessary tools to feel comfortable in creating that opportunity, the beautiful but so rare space, in which we can all feel contained, secure and free to explore the deeper relationship with our experiences, our bodies, and our minds (or our 'bodymindcore'). I thoroughly recommend Noah's informed intuitive approach to anyone wishing to hone their skills in working with their clients in resolving issues with safety and integrity."

—*James Earls, KMI instructor and author of*
Fascial Release for Structural Balance, *Ireland*

"This book challenges us to shift our thinking about the traditional, paternal model of the healing relationship, moving to a deeper and more interconnected perspective. Noah acknowledges the complex personal and interpersonal dynamics involved and guides us to the realization that true healing is only possible in a relationship of collaboration and mutuality. This is an important work that should be considered 'required reading' for any healing profession."

—*Jeff Tarrant, Ph.D., BCN, licensed psychologist, national*
~~eaker and qigong instructor, Columbia, MO

T0186999

"*Getting Better at Getting People Better* is a graceful conversation that expands the notions: practitioner/patron; clinician/client; doctor/patient. Using threads of awareness, Noah weaves a tapestry illuminating trauma and resilience as well as our role as we interact with others. It encourages us to mirror health and breathe."

—*Patricia Pike, speech pathologist, biofeedback/ guided imagery practitioner, Springfield, MO*

"I could perceive and feel the author's well-expressed courage and passion when bringing his critical perception of the interrelationship between practitioner–client. I really like the idea of the two-way system of health, involving both practitioner and client/patron/patient. This book conveys the whole concept very well, with plenty of arguments to make one think or even re-think!"

—*Valeria Ferriera, D.O., London*

"The author gives readers 'THE' tool—their own self!—and explains how to manage, balance and move the energy within. This was a pleasant read for me, inspiring and uplifting too. There is a certain ease to the flow, I did not feel stuck or have to ponder on what was meant, everything was so clear. Clarity in sharing knowledge is such a gleaming quality."

—*Dr. Rupali Jeswal, Healthcare, Rehabilitation and Reintegration, Mumbai, India*

"This book is refreshing, and it's making me look hard at myself as a bodyworker. It has a lot of information that is pertinent for people who give their life to help others but want more than just a how-to book, and want to ponder how perhaps our connection to something more than ourselves is part of the process."

—*Brenda Messling, licensed massage therapist, massage instructor, Fayetteville, AR*

"A must-read for healing professionals interested in creating ethical and reflexive partnerships with their patients. It focuses on the importance of compassionate relationships and self-awareness in providing alternative therapies."

—*Stephanie Norander, Ph.D., Communication, Springfield, MO*

"There is a real call for therapists and counselors to understand the relationship between the emotional body and the physical body, and Noah Karrasch has written a book to help us do just that. Based on his clinical experience and his commitment to helping his clients heal and his students become more effective practitioners, Karrasch has produced an invaluable book, full of practical and enlightening guidance for therapists wanting to learn more about the mind/body connection."

—*Elizabeth Heren, psychotherapist and well-being specialist, London*

"Karrasch invites us to go inside and examine the integrity of the four temples—head, heart, gut and groin, of *both* healing partners. He challenges us to return to the fundamental breath; to complete the inspiration and be aware of the intention of both in and out breaths, looking for that continuous space where health resides. He also suggests how changing words can be pertinent and relevant— 'Too Much Information Syndrome' as a substitute for Trauma, and Emotion seen as energy in motion."

—*Miriam Pessoa Braga, psychotherapist, advanced certified Rolfer, Pilates instructor, Brasilia, Brazil*

"The perspective Noah brings in this book is fascinating as it comes from the heart and combines practical exercises, contemporary theoretical references and a genuine spirit to try to help those who help. Reading this book and applying the suggested approaches in practice brings the healing process to another level."

—*Pedro Prado, Ph.D., psychotherapist and Somatic Experiencing, Advanced Rolfing and Rolf Movement Instructor, Brazil by the same author*

**Freeing Emotions and Energy
Through Myofascial Release**
Foreword by C. Norman Shealy
ISBN 978 1 84819 085 6
eISBN 978 0 85701 065 0

Meet Your Body
**CORE Bodywork and Rolfing Tools
to Release Bodymindcore Trauma**
Illustrated by Lovella Lindsey Norrell
ISBN 978 1 84819 016 0
eISBN 978 0 85701 000 1

GETTING BETTER AT GETTING PEOPLE BETTER

Creating Successful Therapeutic Relationships

Noah Karrasch

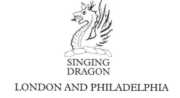

SINGING
DRAGON

LONDON AND PHILADELPHIA

Quote on p.19 from Porges, reprinted by kind permission of Stephen Porges.
Quote on p.31 from Haines 2013, reprinted by kind permission of Steve Haines.
Quotes on p.31 and p.139 from Tolle 2006, reprinted by kind permission of Sounds True.
Quotes on p.47 and p.123 from Taylor 1995, reprinted by kind permission of Kylea Taylor.
Quotes on p.55 from "Presence" by Don Hanlon Johnson, and on p.97 from "Listening to Inner Wisdom" by Shakti Gawain, from *Healers on Healing*, edited by Richard Carlson and Benjamin Shield, copyright © 1989 by Richard Carlson and Benjamin Shield. Used by permission of Jeremy P. Tarcher, an imprint of Penguin Group (USA) LLC.
Quote on p.67 from *In an Unspoken Voice: How the Body Releases Trauma and Restores Goodness* by Peter A. Levine, published by North Atlantic Books, copyright © 2010 by Peter A. Levine. Reprinted by permission of publisher.
Quotes on p.89, p.97 and p.109 from *Care of the Soul in Medicine* by Thomas Moore, copyright © 2010. Reprinted by permission of Hay House, Inc., Carlsbad, CA.
Quote on p.123 from *The Multi-Orgasmic Man* by Mantak Chia and Douglas Abrams Arava. Copyright © 1996 by Mantak Chia and Douglas Abrams Arava. Reprinted by permission of HarperCollins Publishers.
Quote on p.139 from Buckner 2014, reprinted by kind permission of Rod Buckner.
Quote on p.147 from Forni 2002, reprinted by kind permission of Pier Forni.
Quote on p.157 from Steenkamp 2002, reprinted by kind permission of Jo Steenkamp.

First published in 2015
by Singing Dragon
an imprint of Jessica Kingsley Publishers
73 Collier Street
London N1 9BE, UK
and
400 Market Street, Suite 400
Philadelphia, PA 19106, USA

www.singingdragon.com

Copyright © Noah Karrasch 2015

Library of Congress Cataloging in Publication Data
Karrasch, Noah, author.
Getting better at getting people better : touching the core / Noah Karrasch.
p. ; cm.
Includes bibliographical references and index.
ISBN 978-1-84819-239-3 (alk. paper)
I. Title.
[DNLM: 1. Complementary Therapies--psychology. 2. Professional-Patient Relations. 3. Attitude of Health Personnel. 4. Caregivers--psychology. 5. Patient Safety. WB 890]
R733
615.5--dc23
2014013407

British Library Cataloguing in Publication Data
A CIP catalogue record for this book is available from the British Library

ISBN 978 1 84819 239 3
eISBN 978 0 85701 186 2

Printed and bound in Great Britain

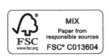

Years ago actress Maureen Stapleton received an Academy Award as Best Supporting Actress. She jumped on stage to deliver this speech:

"I'd like to thank everybody I ever met in my entire life."

Wise woman. She's right—it's the sum of the experiences that make a successful life.

So this book is dedicated to students, patrons, family and friends, but to everybody I ever met in my entire life who helped me shape the thoughts I share.

How do we as practitioners and caregivers learn to deal with our own issues so we can better coax resolution from those seeking energetic balance from us or through us, in our best healing mirror manner? How do we do so in a way that they're enhanced in their self-journey and self-healing and *their desired or chosen self-care and cure? How do we recognize when we, and our patrons, choose to live or hide in various centers of the body, and coax all into the full bodymindcore? This is the conversation offered in* Getting Better at Getting People Better.

ACKNOWLEDGMENTS

Ida Rolf
Emmett Hutchins
Louis Schultz
Stacey Mills
Gil Hedley
Peter Levine
John Sarno
Thomas Moore
Pedro Prado

And readers/critics of early manuscripts:
Bev Breeze, Shiatsu/Watsu
James Earls, Structural Integration
Valeria Ferreira, D.O.
Ralph Harvey, M.D.
Rupali Jeswal, M.D.
Michael Kaufmann, NLP/Reiki
Chris Link, M.D.
Colleen Loehr, M.D.
Peter McGregor, Psychologist/Bodyworker
Brenda Messling, Massage Therapist/Instructor
Stephanie Norander, Ph.D.
Pat Pike, Biofeedback/Guided Imagery
Norm Shealy, M.D., Ph.D.
Jeff Tarrant, Ph.D.

CONTENTS

Prologue   13

1. The Basic Question: Am I Safe?   19

2. Why Are We Sick? Alone, Afraid, Anxious;
   Demoralized or Dead?   31

3. Science vs Intuition   47

4. Which Model Of Healing? Any Model!   55

5. What Gets People Better?   67

   Step 1: Caring   67

   Step 2: Creating safety   75

   Step 3: Communicating   78

   Step 4: Cooperating   83

6. Resolve or Release?   89

7. Physician, Heal Thyself: Embodiment   97

8. Survival: Safety in All its Forms   109

9. Satisfaction Safety   123

10. Self-Esteem Safety   133

11. Purpose Safety   139

12. Clarity Safety   147

13. The Holy Whole Helper: Next Layer   157

APPENDIX A: FOUR AWARENESS EXERCISES TO BRING
ENERGY TO GROIN, GUT, HEART AND HEAD   163

APPENDIX B: TABLES OF OPEN AND CLOSED
PRACTITIONER CENTERS AS THEY RELATE TO OPEN
AND CLOSED PATRON CENTERS   165

REFERENCES   173

INDEX   183

PROLOGUE

This book asks the question of all caregivers, no matter which method or model they follow: *What gets people better, and how can we as helping partners lead them to this better place more fully and more often?* Regardless of the tools we're using, how do we more effectively create and live securely in health and happiness? We want this "better" for our patrons, ourselves, our communities and universes large and small. Finding and holding onto "better's" security may be the big challenge of our century. How do we reclaim feelings of safety as individuals and share them in our society? How do we learn to feel resilient and roll with the punches instead of being sickened by our external challengers?

I'm not a scientist, I'm an observer. I'm not a healer, I'm a helper. I'm not a genius, I'm an intuitive thinker. If I'm a leader, it's possibly because I ask and consider the interesting questions. I've thought at length about the questions of getting better, getting self better, getting others better, and getting community or culture better. I'm personally convinced that if we could more fully discover and truly examine those repressed or unsafe stuck feelings in ourselves, then breathe, and choose to believe in a safe world all around us, we'd have something important to share. We'd be less needed as "healers" and more appreciated as fellow travelers.

I'm able to speak to healing with some authority, having survived a plane crash in 1987 that broke my spine badly at the first lumbar vertebra, a fragile and severe spot to damage. For a while it was doubtful if I'd be able to walk, or function through the lower body again. Due to the bodywork career I'd already embarked on and the thought processes I'd developed over the years regarding how the body, mind and core all work together to produce health or illness, I was able to functionally heal much of my unresolved reaction to this trauma. Let me emphasize that I didn't do this alone! Many people contributed to my healing—which is ongoing, and I'm eternally grateful for all who crossed my path—even those who challenged me in what seemed a negative fashion.

This particular major trauma in my life, and many smaller ones that undoubtedly contributed to both my life problems and their lessons, have served me well. I feel my airplane accident was a major gift in terms of making me a better partner in healing processes. It's my aim to share some of what I've learned through my own experiences, my reactions to these experiences, and my observations of how they impact my patrons in hopes that I can help others become more effective helpers with their clients, patients, patrons and partners in health.

Much of this book is written from the perspective of healing *trauma*. Although one could argue that illness is far different from trauma, and requires a different healing perspective, I offer the concept that actually, old and stored trauma has probably contributed to the emotional state that fosters any illness. We can't unfailingly cure every illness by digging down to find the original emotional trauma and resolve it, but such honest searching will, I believe, contribute to the resolution of illness by simply acknowledging and observing the psychological and physical traumatic roots of that illness.

Years back, I participated in a course on prosperity with my church family. Called the *4T's Program* (for Tithing of Time, Talent and Treasure),[1] it was originated by Stretton Smith and circulated widely in the US Unity church movement. His purpose was to teach us to be more generous and less fearful so as to attract prosperity to ourselves and our world by believing we were *worthy* to receive that very prosperity. Many of his ideas stayed with me, and the following example seems appropriate here.

Stretton asked us to imagine we'd decided to go to a very nice restaurant for an expensive meal. We're seated at our table and admiring the elegance of place settings, décor, attire, patrons, etc.; but begin to wonder why we're being ignored. After several paranoid minutes of watching staff rush to and fro without anyone ever stopping to deliver a menu or even a nod, we finally look across the room to see a large buffet service, and think: "Oh! I've got to get up and get it myself."

I think choosing to be healthy is like that...we've got to ultimately decide that we, the person living in the bodymindcore, will become responsible for our own health. We've got to get up and get it ourselves. There's nothing wrong with asking for help; in fact help is probably essential to achieve health, but it must be both helpful help and wanted help to be effective. If we follow this model, the job of the therapist, practitioner, partner, caregiver, helper, not currently being achieved in too many health-centered relationships, is to share more effectively the needed nutrition our technique and our person offers. We must introduce our client/patient/partner to their own bodymindcore to help them find and feel a satisfied breath in that very core, and also to encourage them to learn and practice a new culture of core accessibility. This wellness is based on feelings of satisfaction...safety, security, satiation. How do we foster and validate for others these feelings of satisfaction if or when *we* can't feel validated or worthy? How do we create fullness all around us, unless we find it for ourselves?

We don't need to make anyone wrong or invalid because they haven't yet found their healthier space, including ourselves. All of us want to be genuine, loving and healthy in most of our thoughts and actions, surrounded by people who want the same. We don't need to try to make others think or feel more like us as we desire to help them. We can't create *for* them the safety of satisfaction, self-esteem, purpose or clarity they need by making them become clones of us. *We want them to get better not for us, but for them.*

We do, when granted permission, get to help them explore their personal core self-awareness: "Look around, see what you like, then get up and feed yourself." It's not our job to "get" people healthy as much as it's our job to help people discover and consider healthy choices. We can show them resilience, but we can't make them resilient. Perhaps we can demonstrate safety, but we can't make them *feel* safe. They've got to get up and get it themselves, but we've got to get better at showing them life's many choices available for consumption. Some choices will make them feel healthy and safe;

others will make them feel unhealthy and fearful. We can learn to be more effective in helping them discern which choices work for them. *We've got to get better at sharing healing* with *others instead of trying to become healers* of *others.*

In *Medicine as Culture: Illness, Disease and the Body*, Deborah Lupton states: "…while we continue to look to medicine to provide help when we are ill, we also sometimes express resentment at the feeling of powerlessness we experience in the medical encounter… In the medical encounter, health-care workers and the patients they are seeking to help must make sense of, interpret and share each other's meanings and assumptions."[2] Which of us hasn't felt some resentment, some feelings of invalidation, when trying to discuss our life with a doctor who's busily trying to get out of the room and down the hall to the next visit, with hopefully a quick restroom trip and several notes of patient visits in between? How can such a caregiver truly care?

The longer I work and the longer I write, the more I'm intrigued by the idea that good health and long life are as simple to achieve as remembering to keep head, heart, gut and groin further apart and in a longer, straighter line. This line allows oneself to *live* in all four spaces contentedly. When we can move cleanly between the four centers and remain grounded in the earth while keeping our heads high, we understand and embody safety of satisfaction, self-esteem, purpose and clarity. These four safeties live in groin, gut, heart and head in my model.

I believe most of us live more fully in one or more of these four centers. Some of us *hide* in one or more of the four. Retrospectively, I believe my first book, *Meet Your Body*,[3] was written for the patron, the person who is often blocked in the groin or gut; for the client in pain who knew it was time to make changes and was willing to get up and get health for him- or herself. The second book, *Freeing Emotions and Energy*,[4] is a heart book, inviting therapists and interested clients to view where their emotional blockages live and how they might begin to free them, and how they can become more effective as "healers" and humans by paying attention to the cues and clues that both their own and their patron's bodymindcore provide.

This third book seems to be coming from and communicating to the head (though it encourages us all to live in all four of the centers, equally)… I'm using no illustrations, I'm quoting far more sources, and I'm working to rise above my own heart-centered world to hopefully close the gap between science and intuition in such a way that both can be served and honored. And, in my head, I'm also interested in helping us as healing partners learn to see those who come to us for help as wounded souls with blocked heads, hearts, guts, groins; one, some or all of these four areas as overactive or underactive. Patrons need direction to find the feast of life that feeds the starving body center(s) and puts the gluttonous one or ones on a diet. I want to challenge us all (*every* healing partner) to learn to open our heads, hearts and guts to our patron-partner-other-mirror-self's groin, gut, heart and head, coaxing forth safety of satisfaction, self-esteem, purpose and clarity—resilience, in them. The groin presents a special challenge, as we all know. We'll talk specifically to that challenge and others as we proceed.

I'm interested in opening the discussion of how every healing modality and practitioner can be more effective by intending to be a healing mirror—not a mechanic, or what I've started thinking of as a "paint-by-number" therapist who can follow the book but can't connect the dots with and to their patrons. How can we as health partners get better at leading our patrons to the buffet and showing them how to feast in a healthy, satisfied and non-indulgent fashion? How do we coax safety and instill resilience merely by our presence and behaviors? How do we get better at encouraging patrons to take charge of their health and their healing, while continuing to explore our own healing path and our own vulnerabilities? How do we refine our skills in sharing healing? And perhaps most important: How do we continue uncovering and renewing ourselves, so we can be better, more effective mirrors for those who cross our path?

I believe if any practitioner allows themselves to seriously consider the content of this book, they can help themselves become better practitioners, as well as fuller and happier people, in service to a greater good. And isn't that ultimately our most important goal?

So, I challenge us all to improve our skills as healing partners. I hope we can learn to assist each other in finding that slow-and-steady out/in/out breathspirit that reaches our tenderest, most painful bodymindcore wounds of anywhichever sort. May we pass through the Valley of the Shadow of Trauma into a higher, self-validating safety of head, heart, gut and groin which restores breath and freshness on the other side—the inside, the core.

CHAPTER 1

THE BASIC QUESTION

AM I SAFE?

...the pivotal point is, can we get people to feel safe?
Stephen Porges[1]

And some of us absolutely don't know how to feel safe on this planet at this time, and have created one of many illnesses, mental, physical or spiritual, as a result of storing that fear in our guts or groins.
Noah Karrasch

As far as I'm concerned, the question above posed by Stephen Porges *is* the basic question. Can we get people to feel safe? Can we admit that when we feel unsafe, our health suffers? Can we consider how to feel safer, and help others find that feeling?

Healing is about balance. Finding healing, and hopefully health as well, is about finding the balance points in oneself that allow one to begin to live in enthusiastic purpose rather than pessimistic endurance, in rich feeling instead of resentful or fearful hiding. In my view we each begin to heal if and when we learn to create and appreciate internal validations instead of seeking external ones. We find resilience—a core readiness and enthusiasm—in our world. We become healthy when we stop bracing ourselves against those external destroyers that can seem to overpower, or have already overpowered any validations, self-esteem or safety on our part. When we can find the personal bodymindcore validation and satisfaction that let us believe and feel we're *good enough*, and when we listen to and operate from that message more of the time, we heal at some deep level. We become truly healthy when we respect ourselves enough to believe we can take care of ourselves and enjoy the process of life.

We've become self-indulgent in our seeking of external validation—satisfaction from without to assuage physical pain or sickness, accidents, emotional rawness, addiction or any other name we give the symptoms of our stresses and stressors. Whether seeking change or trying to prevent or escape it to placate our unhappy souls, we could probably all benefit from allowing ourselves (and allowing others the space to do likewise) to find our inner congestion: our invalidated parts, our vulnerabilities, our wounds, pains and fears. The difficult work consists of knowing how to stay in balance. How do we challenge this pain in ourselves and others without pushing any of us so hard as to bruise and more deeply anchor the old traumas and inner rawness in our bodymindcores? How do we find satisfaction in the moment with our progress, not satisfaction somewhere in the future conditional upon achievement and completion?

Let's not sugar-coat this truth: sometimes healing involves dying, and learning to die peacefully. Too much of medicine currently seems to be based on keeping patients alive at all costs, with quality of life further down the list of desirables. Current statistics[2] suggest 20–40 percent of all health care costs are used to perform unneeded tests. Too much medicine seems to be of the defensive CYA ("Cover Your A---") variety in which medical professionals, intimidated by the threat of being sued for malpractice, order every available test and prescribe medications for simple problems merely to document a paper trail showing they've been "good" doctors. Another large cost in medicine is the unnecessary prolonging of a life that has lost its quality: do we really want to keep Grandma's shell alive at all costs?

A recent *Time Magazine*[3] article dedicated more space to this medical dilemma than to almost any other issue covered in the past few years. This detailed report revealed how hospitals and those who manage them know how to maximize profits at the expense of the unwell, with little regard for the quality of care being delivered. It tells us that 20 percent of our gross domestic product (GDP) is spent on health care. According to author Stephen Brill, "The free market in American medicine is a myth, with or without Obamacare." Something needs to change; we're ready for a more effective model of health. And we've got to get up and get it ourselves. Can we become more effective in our desire to show people that buffet, and help them make healthy choices?

I used interesting terms in the prologue: "sharing healing" and "healing mirrors." I believe that's what true healers do: share healing as well as act as mirrors for their patrons. My model's successful healing relationships are occupied by two individuals who approach a partnership: reflecting, offering, accepting or rejecting, but negotiating opportunities to go into the internal world of one or both partners at a time and endeavoring to release the trapped internal validation, the unhealed trauma of both. Hopefully the practitioner of this healing mirror work has found much of his or her internal awareness, calmness, resilience and mental clarity *before* choosing to be present in mirror partnerships with others. Yet, don't we know that as long as we're on the planet, we're still doing our own healing work? Can we do it with humility and keep our own need for external validation at bay? Such a personality, I think, defines a good practitioner.

I challenge us all to be better healing mirrors for each other. The healing mirror concept suggests that *any* of us, in *any* relationship, can create or facilitate healing simply by providing an honest but loving reflection. Conversely, we can destroy or impede healing if or when we're dishonest and/or judgmental in our reflections—if we present a clouded mirror. If healing relationships don't create health for both parties, perhaps they should be altered or discarded. How clouded is your mirror?

I hope in this book to suggest layers to the healing relationship. First, I don't believe anyone heals anyone else. God heals, nature heals, the higher self heals, the unknown heals, the fill-in-the-blank internal/external power heals. The *inner* heals when the *inner* feels safe and satisfied. The "healer" is merely the conduit or channel through which that goodly/godly type energy emerges and allows healing to occur. I shy away from the term "healer" in this book as much as possible. When designations must be made, "client" and "practitioner" or perhaps better yet, "patron" and "partner" or "helper" and even "seeker" seem appropriate words to me; a *patron* or client supports the concept of health and ultimately gives the stamp of approval to the product or service, while the *helper* assists the patron's choices and the seeker is actually both partners. I've considered substituting the word "other" for "patron," but to me this seems to create a separateness I believe we're seeking to erase. For me, "patron" and "helper" are more complete descriptors for what I want to accomplish with my sessions. I try not to see my patrons as patients or even clients, or myself as a healer instead of a healing mirror, practitioner or helper.

Dr. Ralph Harvey, family practitioner and adjunct faculty member at Michigan State University School of Medicine, suggests to me that "patron" isn't the appropriate word to describe his patient or my client, since it has no connotation of the life-or-death decision the patient often transfers to or shares with their medical authority. This certainly gives me something to ponder as I consider whether I *want* that life-or-death power, or even if I actually want my doctor to take on that much responsibility for me. While a doctor makes life-or-death decisions, we all know the eventual outcome will be death... always. A *patron* chooses to support the healing partner's work; a *patient* is simply too often waiting for something to happen to them, miraculously and patiently.

My colleague Dr. Valeria Ferreira, a Brazilian osteopath, also objects to the term "patron," for linguistic reasons: in Portugese, a *patrao* is a boss, with a connotation of someone who controls others. Yet, shouldn't our clients be in control of their process, and tell us what they want and need?

Thomas Moore, in *Care of the Soul in Medicine*,[4] suggests that, at least in hospitals, a more appropriate designation for "patients" might be "guests." And patrons certainly are paying guests in a hospital! I'm impressed with Moore's desire to change the language around medicine so as to help change medicine itself. When I quote studies or ideas coming from the medical model, I'll echo their language of patient and provider or whichever words they use. Titles aside, *let's remember to co-create a healing relationship* that evokes the innate wisdom of the individual and helps them return to balance without depriving them of control of their own world...even when they want us as "healers" to do exactly that.

Jack Painter, in *Deep Bodywork and Personal Development*[5] gives us this concept clearly: "...all healing is a reciprocal act, and intimate inner and outer contact between the practitioner and individual. Both are taking part in an event which leads toward the balancing of the other's energy—a balance which encourages change and flow of our physical, emotional and mental experience… It may seem that the exchange cannot be equal. After all, you have come to me for help. How can you participate as an equal partner, if part of your armor is a defense against just such an exchange of energy, a resistance at some deep level to the possibility of your own self-transformation? Even if I am centered and initiate my force from inside, and make sensitive, respectful contact with you, but you are afraid to surrender, how can the dance even begin?" How indeed, and how do we get better at initiating the dance and staying in step and in tune with our partners as we show them the feast life can present?

We're still on the planet, so we're still working on our own processes as we work with others. Most of us as practitioners have realized we've sometimes overstepped our bounds, pushed a patron too far, fast or deep, or turned a blind eye to our own frailties, or theirs, in our eagerness to help others. How do we maintain the balance of coaxing satisfaction, self-esteem, purpose and clarity in groin, gut, heart and head—restoring the spirit of the partner—without becoming an addiction for a weak client or patron who simply needs a lifeline, but has no interest in making real changes—the too-patient patient? How do we become something more than placebo? And how do we keep our egos in check so that we don't do *to* these patrons, but encourage them to do *for*, get up and get it, themselves?

And how, how, how do we make them feel safe? How do we foster self-respect and belief in one's own abilities and restore resilience in a world where we're all holding our breath and waiting for the next crisis? In *The Revolutionary Trauma Release Process*[6] David Berceli suggests: "…most of us often tend to run from difficult times, push them away, or pretend they aren't happening. We want to avoid pain and suffering at all cost." And life is becoming ever more difficult. To me the current political, economic and environmental insanities and uncertainties in the US, and around the world, reflect these feelings of unsafety many of us share—be it about bullets coming at us, bullies in our neighborhood, or bullshit from the worlds we've come to accept and even create for ourselves.

Thirty-five years ago I found a book that's been important to me: *Healers On Healing*, compiled by Carlson and Shield,[7] which asked many of the well-known "healers" of that time "What is healing, anyway?" The questioners got some very interesting answers that have provided food for thought over those many years. I'll quote frequently in this book from *Healers On Healing*, since I'm such a fan of what so many successful people had to say. Most of the quotes I've chosen to reproduce are great nutrition in that buffet of life and health. I'm reminded of one such quote in the book, from John Upledger, D.O., founder of the craniosacral school of work, about healing mirrors: "So, the main responsibility of the therapist is to help the patient develop a truer, more correct self-image. This means that when working with a patient, the therapist must become an accurate reflecting mirror, a medium through which the patient's real self can be perceived more clearly."[8] Interestingly, it seems Upledger saw this relationship as a one-way mirror. I think it works both ways, so the patron mirrors for the practitioner as well as vice versa—each partner mirrors for the other.

Everyone is wounded, and all of us carry those traumas— emotional, physical, energetic, chemical, mental, spiritual or other; unless or until someone who cares is sensitive enough to help us move through the painful wounded spot into the pure and unsullied part. In some of us, unsullied is buried very deep. Some of us have become hypersensitized or desensitized and buried our fear or our feelings of a trauma (not even a trauma itself), allowing fear to stop our energy from flowing completely. And some of us absolutely don't know how to feel safe on this planet at this time, and so have created one of many illnesses, mental, physical or spiritual, as a result of storing that fear in our guts or groins, hearts or heads.

Lately another new idea has been forming in me: What if we changed our words, and instead of "trauma," acknowledged "unprocessed information" in our bodymindcores? Can we accept the idea that trauma only becomes trauma when we allow it the space to limit our world, our thinking and our level of pain? Can we realize that everything that comes into us is information, and some information comes too fast, overwhelming us and causing us to store that fear-based feeling deep in the tissues, and leading us to pain, disease and discomfort?

I've long been a fan of Louise Hay, beginning with her books *You Can Heal Your Life* and *Heal Your Body*.[9] In a more recent book, *All is Well*, with Mona Lisa Schulz, Hay emphasizes another important point we must share with our patrons: "The process of identifying the thoughts and behaviors that may be making you ill or making your symptoms worse is not about blaming yourself. You did not cause your illness. Every illness is in part due to factors such as diet, the environment, and genetics. But every illness also can be made worse or better by your emotions."[10] And if your emotions are based in part on that trauma, that unprocessed information, how can we learn to resolve that unfinished business?

I've also recently been absorbing John Sarno's book, *The Divided Mind*.[11] Among the most interesting ideas Sarno presents, I first resonate with his sense that "psychosomatic" isn't necessarily a "dirty" word. We needn't assume someone is stupid, bad or a malingerer because they acknowledge their difficulties have psychosomatic roots. He contends every condition in the physical body probably does have emotional threads which contribute, if not outright cause, the condition one wants to change. Sarno has labeled the trauma many of us experience as "Tension Myositis Syndrome" (TMS). He suggests that much of what goes wrong in our world, be it carpal tunnel syndrome, post-traumatic stress disorder or fibromyalgia, to name a few, can be traced to our inability to respond appropriately to the traumas that pervade our lives. He argues that many of these diseases could have been around for years (carpal tunnel? We've been typing for years...why now? PTSD? People have been going to war for years...why now? Fibromyalgia? Traumatic incidents have attacked people for years...why now?). It's an interesting, thought-provoking argument.

When Sarno diagnoses TMS, his evaluation nearly always finds a personality that is either "perfectionist" or "goodist." These people try to do for others at their own expense, and end up in pain because they repress their true feelings. "...the altered physiology in TMS appears to be a mild, localized reduction in blood flow to a small region or a specific body structure, such as a spinal nerve, resulting in a state of mild oxygen deprivation…the true cause of the pain, TMS, serves the purpose of *primary gain*, that is, to prevent the conscious brain from becoming aware of unconscious feelings like rage or emotional pain."[12] Feeling pain is easier than feeling feelings!

Lately I've been thinking to myself that perhaps we could even simplify life and create and use the term TMIS—"Too Much Information Syndrome." It seems we all multi-task so much in our effort to keep up, look busy, achieve more and feel better about who we are and what we do, that we drive ourselves into sickness and pain with our efforts. We allow too much information to reside in our bodymindcore and can't keep it all straight. This overwhelm contributes to our pain and causes us to be less satisfied in our lives. We can identify this condition as too much information or as trauma; either asks us to focus more positively on release and resolution.

So I suggest we can become better healing partners by first acknowledging the emotional component to many patrons' problems—their fear of facing the unknown. This book encourages us to help others become more resilient and more self-aware as they process their trauma's information. I put forth the practitioner as healing mirror, willing to seek and accept healing of self in the process of working with others. I encourage in *both* healing partners the recognition and expression of the woundedness and fear of living most of us feel, so healing can occur. I share thoughts and themes designed to examine healing relationships, with appropriate comments from others I admire and respect for their healing presence and talents.

Our job then, simply and profoundly I think, is to *create and maintain effective therapeutic relationships between practitioner and patron—* the practitioner's responsibility and, ultimately, their measure of success. How do we support safety and resilience without becoming a patron's new drug of choice? What makes some therapeutic relationships successful, while others fail? Is there a way to predict with whom and how success will occur? Can we learn from our practitioner mistakes so that the next patron will receive the challenge, the healing, the resolution in the appropriate dosage, and move on with life effectively and freely? Why do some therapists seem to have "it" while others continue to struggle to attract clients and to help those they attract? I'm intrigued by those questions, and think there's much to reflect on here for all of us, regardless of therapeutic setting or model.

Like most allopathic practitioners, many alternative caregivers fall into the trap of believing they're supposed to "fix" a client's problems and magically make symptoms disappear. Often this very therapist is the one who, perhaps unknowingly, went into a helping profession simply to work on their own process through the clients' stories or bodies... Too often they're truly working to repair client issues as a way of salving and solving their own problems. Perhaps their breakthrough in a mode of therapy revealed its value to them so strongly that they felt called to participate in that healing profession. It's good that we as therapists believe in our own tools; it's damaging to clients when we choose to see our model as the only effective tool in the toolkit that's our personal therapeutic brand, or when we label a client as difficult simply because they don't respond to who we are and what we have to offer. Every practitioner and technique is right for someone; no practitioner or technique is right for everyone. How do we more effectively match the appropriate technique and helper to the appropriate client/patron, in the appropriate dosage, and how do we make our technique and presence right for more of the people who come to our studios, clinics or offices?

Quite a few of us, both in and out of the traditional medical community, have had difficulties or differences with the current allopathic medical establishment. Often these problems are brought on, I believe, by our negative reactions to the profit motive that's present too much of the time. I want us all to make a living wage, and indeed a healthy living wage. I'm not a fan of "non-profit" medical centers which have to justify their profits, so reinvest in larger state-of-the-art buildings and equipment or swallow small independent clinics, without bothering to expend energy to teach their doctors or nurses to spend time listening to those who come through their doors. I don't understand why these places don't better appreciate and reward the aides and orderlies who spend the most time with patients in a truly caring fashion. By taking a bit less profit, hospitals could reward those who interact with patients, provide better care for them, re-personalize medicine, and make a healthier system for all of us. And better yet, they could charge their patients less money!

I think many of us agree that greed is rampant in our world, not just in the medical system, but through the very fiber of society. The basic question returns in another form: Are the greediest in all walks merely unhealthy people trying to create safety in their own worlds? Are they seeking satisfaction instead of being satisfied? Can we truly get well, or deliver health and wellness in such a greed-based world?

I'm reminded of a recent research project by Abrams, Dolor, Roberts *et al.* from the journal *Complementary and Alternative Medicine*,[13] which showed substantial improvement in quality of life and overall wellbeing among patients who used complementary medicine in addition to their prescribed medical treatments. Over six months these patients showed less depression, less severe pain, and in general were more satisfied with their treatment and progress. It's happening. Patients are waking up to the idea that they should be part of the healing team.

My first career was music; I taught school music in the US for five years here and there, and played piano and sang in clubs and restaurants for another ten. One night early in my career, when I was singing what I considered to be my best original work, the last patron left the bar during my special song. I realized I was missing some important connection to my patrons. This realization led me to learn to be an entertainer, and to realize that merely presenting my best stuff wouldn't necessarily engage the patron. I saw clearly that involving the patron and seeking participation from them was the key to creating a satisfying experience for us all. That important lesson about entertaining/selling to my patrons has never left me. I feel it applies to being a true caregiving, healing partner mirror. Some might see this as a "fake-it-'til-you-make-it" attitude, but I see it as common sense. I do want to involve my patrons, because I do care about their experience with me. And the more I care about them, the more they feel that caring and the more fully they respond.

In this book we'll examine less specifically the individual techniques or modalities we may know and use, and focus more on the generalities of what gets people better and how to apply these generalities to our own particular healing work more effectively. We'll keep our guiding question in mind: Can we get people to feel safe? We'll think about what's working in the current system, but also what isn't, and we'll focus on creating healing relationships instead of power relationships.

It's my intention to provoke thought in other interested caregivers as I work to enhance and improve my own partner skills for my patrons in our processes. I'm not yet "there," or I wouldn't even need to write this book. I believe I teach what I need to learn, and I constantly work to enhance my own skills. We're all learning, all the time—or should be. When we stop learning about our own tools, our own process, and our own ability to relate more effectively to others, it's time to pull down the shingle and find another pastime. If you're interested in questioning your effectiveness as a healing mirror practitioner partner, no matter whether in a professional setting or in a personal relationship, there may be something for you in the following chapters. And if you're simply interested in feeling better about what you do and who you are as a practitioner, please read on, with an open mind and heart.

CHAPTER 2

WHY ARE WE SICK?

ALONE, AFRAID, ANXIOUS; DEMORALIZED OR DEAD?

Dissociation is part of the body's response to overwhelming stress.
Steve Haines[1]

What is the real arch enemy of the little me? The present moment.
Echkart Tolle[2]

*These people want to get better, and I need to get
better at helping them find their way.*
Noah Karrasch

People get sick when they feel unsafe, unsure, unloved or unenthusiastic about life. They lose self-respect when they realize they can't cope with life as it's playing out around them. They don't know how to turn off those less-than feelings, turn them around or shake them out to become enthused and alive again. Slowed-down emotional energy slows down the physical energies as well. This thought makes one of Louise Hay's affirmations seem even more appropriate: "I am willing to feel. It is safe for me to express my emotions. I love myself."[3]

Years ago, I met my first client with fibromyalgia. At the time little was known about the condition (and still is, truthfully). We're now deciding it's a condition of extremely inflamed nerves, but unsure exactly what to do about that condition, or why the nerves are inflamed. I found my early clients with fibro presented a special challenge to me as I didn't know how to touch them appropriately, how to get through their defenses, and how to help them move forward. For a good while, I decided there was something about the fibro personality that suggested to me they didn't want to get better. Eventually, my realization came: These people want to get better, and I need to get better at helping them find their way. Once I had that shift in my thinking, fibro clients indeed began to improve dramatically. This speaks to an important point, I think, *and* feel.

I've long been a fan of teaching patrons and students, and myself, to remember to breathe more deeply, fully and often. I've come to believe that fibromyalgia is a disease of "I've had the wind knocked out of me and I can't catch my breath." By that criterion, most of us could be said to suffer from fibro in some form or degree. Most of us are stuck in our breath somewhere—either waiting to exhale, forgetting to inhale or just holding our breath.

It may be this fibromyalgia plague of our times is caused simply by the inability to remember to breathe in and out, gently, slowly, uniformly, often due to our response to life's traumas. This new plague could be and has been identified in many ways: panic or anxiety, fibromyalgia, post-traumatic stress disorder, repetitive motion disorders or, as Sarno calls the condition, "Tension Myositis Syndrome (TMS), a painful psychosomatic disorder afflicting millions."[4] To me, *all* diagnoses are signals that something has taken away one's ability to breathe.

If we subscribe to the concept that the world feels unsafe to most of us, you can see why we might hold our breath. Perhaps it's as simple as trying to keep at bay unresolved childhood abuse issues that caused one to try to be invisible *back then*, but keep one hiding in the *now*. Perhaps it's absorbing too much news and feeling unsafe in one's neighborhood or world. Perhaps it's enduring a relationship where one feels unheard, misunderstood or threatened. For whichever of many reasons (nearly as many reasons as there are people on the planet), too many of us are afraid to take a deep and cleansing breath.

Recently a bodywork student in one course asked me what I know of people who seem to be locked at the top of an inhale— what I'd call an "inspired" person. His question was, what do we do to help them? My answer is simple: Teach them to inhale, but also to exhale. This led me to remember that many people are what I think of as "expired" people; those who never bother to bring any air in beyond a small and essential minimum. Again, we must teach clients, and self, to breathe!

I worked briefly with a new patron who's had good bodywork from many sources. Yet after many sessions this man had no concept of how to breathe, so hadn't made much progress towards releasing or resolving the tension in his body. In one session, I quickly saw his inbreath reached only to a count of two. As I worked with him, I coaxed him into longer breaths, with little success. Finally, deciding he was an achiever, I challenged him to bring in breath to a count of five instead of two. It worked! Fairly quickly, he learned to take long, nurturing inhales and exhales, which he'd not bothered to do in the recent past. We made remarkable progress in one hour, predicated on his learning to breathe in and out.

Dr. Ralph Harvey recently told me about the work he's tracking with alternative techniques.[5] He's recently found that slow and regular breathing, which is to say six breaths per minute, brings down sympathetic nerve tone and allows the parasympathetic tone to rise. This in turn sends signals to the vagus nerve to relax (we'll return to examine the vagus a bit later). One outcome of slow, focused and regular breathing is increased heart rate variability (HRV). Increase in HRV can be seen as a marker for other body changes…like overall decrease in inflammation. It's also associated with improved cardiac function, relaxed brainwave patterns, decrease in LDL bad cholesterol, decrease in stress hormones and decreased inflammatory disorders.

Think of nearly any condition in the body that's problematic, and realize that a good breath might just be the beginning of correcting the underlying cause of the problem! I've long tried to convince my patrons to learn to expand their breath capacity and their ability to exchange oxygen by breathing out even longer than they breathe in. For example, if they can breathe in for a count of 8, I invite them to try to breathe out for a count of 12, which ensures cleansing of the lungs.

Peter Levine in *In an Unspoken Voice*[6] offers this clue to breath's importance: "Breathing that is rapid, shallow and/or high in the chest indicates sympathetic arousal. Breathing that is very shallow (almost imperceptible) frequently indicates immobility, shutdown, and dissociation."

Many of us are taking shallow breaths because we're either still afraid of something (fighting or fleeing), or because we've decided to freeze up our bodies until the danger has passed—even though we probably no longer know what the danger even is or was!

Levine discusses, in *Trauma-Proofing Your Kids* with Maggie Kline,[7] the concept of *resilience*, which I might define as "a relaxed yet dynamic bodymindcore that believes in its power to cope with life's challenges." He calls resilience "...the capacity we all possess to rebound from stress and feelings of fear, helplessness and overwhelm." He argues that we all receive trauma (remember, we can think of trauma as unprocessed information), and wonders why some of us are able to shake out trauma and move forward while others get anchored in our traumas and can't release or resolve them, so end up bearing them, internally and alone. He suggests openness is the characteristic that resilient people share. How do we foster openness in our patrons? Perhaps it's as simple as teaching them to remember to breathe and exhale the trauma. Perhaps best yet, we can abandon the concept of trauma and substitute "information" or "stimulus"; then breathe to release this stimulus.

A new school of work is presently developing: Trauma Informed Care.[8] This work encourages the realization that most of us who have been exposed to trauma would like to release it but, critically, must first learn to feel safe again. This style seems to resonate with Levine and Porges in their belief in the creation of safety as the first step to true healing. And remember my idea that trauma can be seen as too much information or stimulation; how do we process it all?

Berceli[9] shares this distinction about stress, anxiety and trauma: "Stress comes from the feeling that a certain set of circumstances should not be happening... Anxiety stems from the feeling that something should be happening that clearly isn't... In both stress and anxiety, our inner experience is that we want to be somewhere other than where we are... What's happening is that something in the present has triggered unprocessed trauma from the past, and this is now emerging as distress." We become stressed when we can't control *what's happening* to us, and anxious when we can't control *what's not happening* to us. Both stress and anxiety contribute to us revisiting our memory files to find what we consider to be an appropriate response to any current stimulus or trauma, based on a past response to a past trauma that was possibly never properly resolved.

A study by Orlinsky and Howard in 1986[10] concluded that openness or self-relatedness, even defined as selfishness, was found to be a personality trait consistently related to a positive outcome in therapy. What this study suggests to me is that I've got to get better and better as a caregiver in learning how to coax openness, self-relatedness, even selfishness, and known and felt safety from my patron by demonstrating it in myself. This is a key aspect of helping to create self-respect and security in clients and patrons. When we can make a safe place for them to express who they really are and what's truly bothering them, we've given them the gift of space in which to acknowledge and heal their hurts. They're no longer alone or afraid or anxious. They can breathe again! They're then able to be resilient and have a chance to release and resolve whichever traumas have managed to become embedded in them.

I've long cited Jerome and Julia Frank's book, *Persuasion and Healing*,[11] in which they suggest research shows four commonalities that effective healers/therapists display. First, the client needs to feel the therapist *really cares about them and their life*; this instills some of the external validation and fosters the openness we all crave. Second, the *treatment setting is nurturing and safe* and the client can therefore achieve the gut-level honesty, the self-relatedness with themselves and their partner practitioner, the fulfilling exhale, without fearing judgment. Third, *the therapy model is communicated, understood* enough to allow the client to believe in the possibility of the model, *and respected by both partners*. The client can enthusiastically get on board with a process they understand and trust. Fourth, and arguably most important, *the client is expected to participate in their process* as a doer rather than a done-to. They've got to get up and get it themselves. When these four boxes are ticked, honestly, clients respond and get better, regardless of the model of therapy being offered. These four points will be discussed more fully in Chapter 5.

This simple yet profound score card offers us much to ponder. We're all aware of partner practitioners who fall down on one or more of these points. An unprofessional setting and uninviting demeanor, or a space that doesn't allow the patron to let down their guard, to unwind and release or resolve issues, isn't conducive to change. People who hold their breath won't get well. Poor communication about the process to and from patrons who expect to be healed with a magic pill or surgery, without discussing details like their own investment in the healing process, often produces substandard results or no results at all. Quite simply, if we subscribed to these four truths and made them our goals more diligently, remembering to check our therapeutic skills against the four boxes, our success rate (in terms of both numbers of patrons and success with them) would probably increase.

Persuasion and Healing remains a textbook for what works in therapies. In addition to the above four-part formula, one other aspect of this book rings true for me. The Franks suggest illness is caused by "demoralization." "Regardless of their training, healers may be effective if they are able to combat patients' demoralization, mobilize their expectation of help, and shore up or restore their self-confidence."[12]

In other words, when we lose our purpose in life, when we can't find our joy, when energy or juice doesn't flow through us, we become afraid, anxious, demoralized and sick. Maybe we become sick because we're afraid; maybe we become afraid because we're sick. Either makes us feel alone, isolated, different and less-than. While this seems to be common sense, too many times I think we as practitioners forget this simple truth. What gets someone enthused? Is there anything in life that makes them happy, makes them want to bravely and enthusiastically continue with it? Can we find, or help them find, that key to "re-morale-ize" them so they can catch their breath? Can we help them find their internal validation and wean them from the need for external validators? Can we help them become more resilient, more core-relaxed, to allow their feelings to flow through instead of getting stuck in their bodymindcores? Is this the "self-relatedness" described above by Orlinsky and Howard?

I'm also reminded of an idea from *The Human Element* by Will Schutz.[13] In a book devoted to examining what makes groups work well, or poorly, he begins with the idea that lack of self-esteem is the root cause of too many problems we have in our lives. In this theory he echoes Louise Hay, who's been suggesting for years that at the root of most illnesses can be found feelings of low self-esteem. Schutz says: "The ramifications of high or low self-esteem are enormous and ubiquitous, and their extent is often underestimated. They affect every aspect of human personality and human interaction. They affect our productivity and ability to think creatively and logically. They are often the source of our social problems… In fact, the most I can do for any other person is to help him or her become fully realized. I can do that only when I myself am unafraid and open." Well! There's the challenge. Fully realized, self-related, resilient or re-morale-ized…how do we achieve that feeling of safety and satisfaction, of "good enough-ness" so we demonstrate it to and coax it from our patrons? How can we help them release what's taken their breath away from them?

Schutz and Hay are seconded by Twerski in *Addictive Thinking: Understanding Self-Deception*:[14] "A person can feel bad or worthless, even though this is a total contradiction to reality. Feeling insecure and inadequate makes a person more vulnerable to escapism, so often accomplished via mood-altering drugs. The person feels different from the rest of the world, as if he or she doesn't belong anywhere… Many thinking distortions are not necessarily related to chemical use. For example, fear of rejection, anxiety, isolation, and despair often result from low self-esteem. Many of the quirks of addictive thinking are psychological defenses against these painful feelings." Feelings based on insecurity and lack of safety result in lack of health and shortness of breath. And we return to resilience; those who maintain self-esteem worry far less about what the world might think of them, and are better able to deal with life in each moment, instead of hiding from life in every moment.

Sarno again: "It is my view, as it was Adler's, that *feelings of inferiority* are universal, varying in degree and intensity, but not limited to 'neurotics'… The drive to be perfect and good are reactions to feelings of inferiority, which are always unconscious (and sometimes conscious as well). Such tendencies to achieve and be nice are typical of people trying to demonstrate by their performance and behavior that they are worthwhile, not inferior."[15] One of Sarno's followers, Andrea Leonard-Segal says this even better: "Getting better from TMS is learning how to extract yourself from needing recognition from others and learning how to fill that need yourself…about learning that almost all of the time that you feel guilty, it is inappropriate, in that you cannot be responsible for taking care of everyone's feelings."[16]

I've previously quoted Stephen Porges, who has spent the past 30 years researching the vagus nerve, its functions and scope, and has developed a "polyvagal theory."[17] He theorizes that the vagus nerve, which I think of as the center of well-being, and which others call the "anti-stress" mechanism, is more important than we've thought. We might even suggest the vagus nerve creates feelings of resilience and core relaxation, *the* overall coping skill that can keep us healthy (or, in its absence, make us ill). He suggests it not only regulates circulation and digestion as it moves from the head, through the neck and down the front of the spine, but also controls both a great deal of relaxation response *and* the adrenal fight-or-flight response. The very name "vagus" suggests the word vague…indeed, this is a vague nerve. It travels from the neck, the only cranial nerve to reach down into the lower body. It serves the heart, lungs, liver, stomach, kidneys, adrenals and intestines. We truly don't know the extent of its abilities, I believe. We're not exactly sure what it does, but we know its effects are felt everywhere. And remember Dr. Harvey's realization (see page 33) that slow and even breath increases heart rate variability, which in turn allows for healthier vagus function.

Porges' polyvagal approach speculates that the vagal/adrenal system has an older, earlier channel beyond fight-or-flight. This channel brings us yet another survival mechanism, which could be called the "freeze" or "play dead" response. Perhaps you've witnessed a cat playing with a mouse; perhaps this mouse, while being challenged, automatically went into a "play dead" response until the threat of the cat was gone. When the cat no longer sees sport in the play, the mouse will "come to" and scamper away.

Like lower animals, we have this older, internal play dead system, which we use to our detriment because of the amount of stress and unsafety we absorb in our lives. Porges tells us 90 percent of the fibers in this nerve are afferent fibers, which is to say, fibers returning from the body to the brain. Only ten percent of our vagus fibers are motor fibers that run from the brain to the body, efferently. This means that our true brain really does in some ways reside in our gut! For every nerve fiber that sends commands to the body, there are nine fibers sending information back to the brain about how the body is responding to the brain's commands. This suggests we are governed by our feelings more than by our thought! Autonomically we move; our thoughts follow our bodies, not the other way around.

I have a memory of my first play dead experience… I was perhaps ten years old, and my best friend was a year older and five inches taller. One day on the schoolyard, he grabbed me from behind in a bear hug. Without thinking, I bent forward, flipping him over my body. He immediately jumped up, angry that a smaller child had shamed and bested him, and proceeded to beat me. I curled into a ball and allowed him to pummel, push, roll and do whatever he wanted until his anger was spent, at which point he walked away and I came back to life. Only in retrospect can I see this as my first remembered experience of freezing to avoid something unpleasant or life-threatening. By going limp, I was able to avoid much of the abuse he would have heaped on me if I'd resisted. Something in me went primal and avoided more abuse.

The central nervous system (CNS) travels through the spinal cord, innervating much of the body. This older vagal system of autonomic nerve function automatically responds to our thoughts even before we know we've had them! How do we become more aware in this system, so that we more quickly develop the resilience that allows us to live more fully in our bodymindcores?

Sarno echoes Porges' thought: "…it is emotions that drive the chemistry in the brain, not the other way around. Altered serotonin chemistry is not a disorder, it is an emotionally induced chemical reaction resulting from the true symptom, which is depression."[18] An interesting concept: our chemicals change in response to our thoughts, not the other way round.

Porges reiterates that as healing practitioner partners, one of our greatest challenges is to help our patrons feel safe and learn to remain in feelings of safety. Thus our chapter's title makes sense: Whether alone, afraid, anxious, demoralized or playing dead, we've stopped breathing and it's made us sick. The creation of safety can stimulate the bodymindcore to engage the newer circuits of the nervous system that create calm and self-soothing. When on alert, we move into the fight-or-flight response with older and deeper fibers, and if necessary, we move into the freeze response through the oldest vagal system.

Much of Porges' research is being done with post-traumatic stress disorder (PTSD) and autistic populations, which may both be groups of extremely unsafe-feeling people. But his question seems to fit any unhealthy or unfulfilled population: "…the pivotal point is, can we get people to feel safe?"[19] Levine might phrase the question thus: "Can we get people to find their inner resilience?" Interestingly, a recent study shows that PTSD sufferers who have taken up running are often being released from its symptoms.[20] Perhaps it's the movement of the body's tissues back into and through the trauma; perhaps it's because that movement both fosters resilience and releases endorphins.

For me as a bodywork practitioner partner, when the patron feels unsafe, this freeze or play dead response can be demonstrated in many forms. Some folks don't seem to live in their bodies at all. They have no sense of pain when they're being touched—or, conversely, every touch is nearly too painful to be endured. Some chatter incessantly to take their mind off the experience the body is receiving—and not just during their bodywork sessions. Some power past the pain, and perhaps hold their breath until the unaware practitioner finally lets go of the already-traumatized, and now freshly-damaged bodymindcore. Some simply stop breathing at any discernible level (if they were even breathing when they arrived). Some even fall asleep. All these coping mechanisms could be seen as forms of the older vagal response to a stressful situation—a freezing or playing dead to escape the actual confrontation of that which feels unsafe.

Shouldn't there be some sort of position on the gauge of adrenal response that approximates to "neutral"? If fight represents facing trauma (perhaps fearfully, but with committed life force), flight represents running, fearfully, from it. Freeze represents hiding, fearfully. Could *feel* represent exploring, consciously, our traumas or any of life's stimuli, and the way we're processing them, without fear? Can we learn to live with our gauges set on "feel" instead of "fight," "flee," or "freeze"? Health comes from understanding how much of the external world represents potential trauma and dealing with it more quickly. We're sick because we're defending our core against our environment. We become healthier by deciding to see each potential from the outside as an opportunity to receive and process outside information, instead of a need to defend against it.

As Jo Steenkamp, author of *SHIP* (Spontaneous Healing Intrapersonal Process) says, "Pain…means that there is a part of me that still *needs* to express itself… The only diagnosis I believe we can justifiably make is one of a chronic systemic stress reaction, in which the client is the healer and the carrier of internal wisdom."[21] Steenkamp further suggests the use of the term "EBlock," representing "emotions in myself blocking me." Interestingly, I've always thought the word "emotion" could be seen as a shorthand term for "energy in motion." When energy isn't in motion, but stifled because of blocks in the system, we have a recipe for illness.

This work echoes Peter Levine's groundbreaking book *Waking the Tiger*.[22] Levine posits that we all hold on, freeze in response to stress, and have forgotten how to feel and process our feelings. Thus, we're nearly walking dead. He encourages us to learn to retrieve feelings, express them, move through them and get on with our lives.

Sarno calls the condition "Tension Myositis Syndome" (see page 32). David Berceli, creator of the Trauma Release exercises, maintains, "Every trauma, whether it occurs in a physiological, cognitive, emotional or interpersonal form, affects the physical body."[23] Berceli suggests that a traumatic reaction isn't a negative response, but a positive one—an attempt by the body to protect itself. He therefore sees the shaking response in both bodywork and mental work as a good thing, a release of old trauma stored deep in the bodymindcore.

Eckhart Tolle adds to this discussion in *New Earth: Awakening to Your Soul's Purpose*: "Because of the human tendency to perpetuate old emotion, almost everyone carries in his or her energy field an accumulation of old emotional pain, which I call the 'pain-body'… Any negative emotion that is not fully faced and seen for what it is in the moment it arises does not completely dissolve. It leaves behind a remnant of pain… Any emotionally painful experience can be used as food by the pain-body...The pain-body is an addiction to unhappiness."[24]

Scott Peck, in *People of the Lie,* asks a pertinent question: *"...do people see a psychiatrist because their problems are greater than average or because they possess greater courage and wisdom with which to face their problems more directly?"*[25] Do some of us, feeling unsafe, choose to take the leap into that unsafe place and over the dreaded chasm to find the joy on the other side, while others stay on the bank, fearful of even attempting the leap? Do some seek help only because they can't control or cope with symptoms on their own, while others have the courage to find and cope with a healing partner and the attendant negotiations? Can we recognize where on the path each individual is and assist them in their journey, without confusing their journey by asking them to walk our path?

I've long resonated with a thought I've heard from several sources, including Rachel Naomi Remen and Christiane Northrup,[26] who suggest that illness can be seen as a form of meditation... If we don't allow our bodymindcore time to relax and unwind, eventually we may just create some opportunity that gives us that down time! We're simply giving ourselves a much-needed rest.

Some practitioners seem to know naturally how to tick the Franks' four boxes (caring, creating safety, communicating and cooperating— see page 36), help others find the self-esteem highlighted by Hay and Schulz, coax them to release repressed feelings, as Sarno and Steenkamp suggest, create Porges' safety in their sessions, or induce Berceli's or Levine's trauma release. Others seem to fall down in one or more of the Franks' four areas. Whichever model is used, if the patron feels they are a full participant with a practitioner who lets them know what, and in many cases why something is happening and *how they can be helpful,* either before or during the session, more is achieved.

Doctors are often cited for poor communication skills; studies have shown that doctors with good communication abilities are subjected to fewer malpractice lawsuits. In one study, 42 percent of malpractice claims reflected communication breakdowns.[27] Yet communication with patients is only beginning to be taught in many medical schools.

Too many schools still seem to follow the old dictum that doctors can't get close to patients because "if you care about them, you'll be disappointed when you lose them." Doctors therefore must withhold a part of self and continue to pretend to have knowledge that none of us can truly have in every situation. It's hard to help someone feel less alone, afraid or anxious if you don't know how to talk with them. We'll spend more time with these thoughts in Chapter 5.

And here, I'd add one thought that comes through many practitioners, but is perhaps best summarized by Peter Levine:[28] "My experience…working with so many more traumatized clients, has taught me that the very key to resolving trauma is being able to *uncouple and separate the fear from the immobility*… Kahlbaum had it right when, in 1874, he wrote, 'In most cases catatonia is *preceded* by grief and anxiety, and in general by depressive moods and affects aimed against the patient by himself'…the therapist's job is to aid a client to gradually uncouple the fear from the paralysis, so as to gradually restore self-paced termination… Too much, too soon, threatens to overwhelm the fragile ego structure and adaptive personality. This is why the rate at which people resolve trauma must be gradual and 'titrated.'" In other words, a reagent must be *carefully* introduced in the proper dosage to cause (hopefully healing) change in the situation/ substance/person. How do we get better at separating our patrons from their problems and bringing them back to "alive"?

Frank and Frank have this to say about their use of the term "demoralization": "For many people the distress of a crisis or social breakdown is compounded by the feeling that they are somehow unique, that no one else has ever been through a similar experience, and that therefore no one really understands them…to the extent that a patient's symptoms are expressions of demoralization, restoration of self-esteem by whatever means may cause the symptoms to subside."[29] Too many of us become demoralized because of an idea, a trauma, or a thought of a trauma—a chance innocent remark or a truly evil action from an outside other can crush the spirit of health that lives in all of us and destroy the fragile safety and satisfaction we've found. How do we as practitioner partners reach in and coax people out of that demoralized place and into the full stream of life again, with effective and caring communication? That's where healing lies.

I've alluded to the idea that some ill or traumatized people never actually experience a deep physical or emotional trauma. An offhand remark can set a person on an unhealthy path which was never envisioned by the person who made the comment. Some people are so sensitive, so *non*-resilient, that the *threat* of a perceived trauma has triggered them to shut down—to flee or freeze, perhaps to fight, but usually to *not* feel. In some way, they're trying to control their world even as they realize it's not the world they want. As healing partner practitioners we want to help them experience safety so they can review the old physio-emotional conditioning that's caused them to shut down. We can then help them realize they can release that old conditioning and its established coping mechanisms and resolve the condition by replacing old patterns with a healthier, more appropriate and more energetic pattern, so as to live a re-morale-ized life.

Viktor Frankl, in *Man's Search for Meaning*[30] sheds light on this situation effectively. A World War II concentration camp survivor, Frankl, as a psychiatrist, became determined to stay busy in the camp by observing the behaviors of prisoners around him. He noted that prisoners who found a purpose for living, did so. It could be a very negative reason to be alive: seeking revenge, expressing anger or grief. It could be a positive goal: reuniting the family, retrieving a hidden fortune, moving on with life. No matter what the reason for staying alive, those who found and clung to their purpose were often able to survive the horrors of the camps; those who couldn't find a reason to survive, didn't. Those who could keep their heart in it, kept their heart beating. The demoralized gave up on life, while those who re-morale-ized themselves and found internal validation stayed alive, even in an unsafe world.

So why are we sick? Alone, afraid, anxious, demoralized or dead? The reason may be as simple as low self-esteem, inappropriate response to triggers that cause us to shrink, lack of resilience, or demoralization. It may be that we suffer from TMS, TMIS, PTSD, fibro or some other painful condition that relates to our own repression of who we are or who we want to be. All seem to point to an internal fear or holding that takes our breath away. Perhaps the next question should be: Are any of these conceptual disorders possible to understand and treat effectively? If so, how? Let's move further into what can make us well, with a slight detour to look at the duality of science and intuition.

CHAPTER 3

SCIENCE VS INTUITION

As a midwife to the psychospiritual developmental process
occurring in nonordinary states, the therapist permits, protects,
and ushers forth that which wants to happen of its own accord.

Kylea Taylor[1]

I'm asking those with scientific minds not to let go of
their need for science and knowledge, but to suspend their
negative judgment of intuition and consciousness.

Noah Karrasch

Lately I've been paying attention to many in various health care communities—both allopathic and alternative medicine—who demand more and more "evidence-based" technique. They contend that unless one can say exactly what a technique does in a specific bodymindcore situation to the person and their problem, and *why* it's working, it's not a valid technique. These people basically say, "Show me the data." They believe if one can't duplicate or replicate results from client to client, the technique is flawed.

For me, that worldview is flawed! I see us all as individuals in process; more and more I have a hard time trying to put all who come through my door into the same mold or model which seeks to guarantee a result. I'm frustrated by students who want me to teach specific techniques in a "one-size-fits-all" mode, just as much as they're frustrated by my inability to give such specifics. I think of working with each patron in the same way, with exactly the same set of guidelines, as "paint-by-number" bodywork. I perceive myself as an artist, not a technician. I've been challenged by those who discount the validity of intuition, or insight, or spirituality, or whatever word one might use to describe that unscientific interaction and relationship that can be created with the patron. The idea that a practitioner partner wants to rely on science exclusively seems as wrong to me as the idea that I as a helper should rely on intuition exclusively, without having any science behind me. I've studied my anatomy (as have most serious artists), but I often allow my hands and heart to tell me what to do with my patrons, based on scientific *and* intuitive knowledge.

In 1985 I attended the first Comprehensive Studies program at the Rolf Institute in Boulder, Colorado, a program designed to give non-massage-oriented students a preparatory course for Rolf training. Among our professors was James Oschman,[2] researcher, scientist, author and thinker. His first lecture has always rung true for me. He challenged us to consider that much of what is seen as scientific fact is simply the best story some thinker has yet created. Just as all used to believe the archaic idea that the earth was flat, most of us choose to believe a certain idea, then go and seek our data to support our thesis—since people long ago couldn't see a curved surface, they assumed the earth was flat. However, after someone collected enough data, they convinced others to believe the round-earth theory, and it has become accepted scientific fact—until someone comes along with a better story. Perhaps science will one day determine the earth is actually a hologram and we're not even here! It seems to me that Oschman's thesis all too often proves to be true.

Oschman is supported by scientist and author Samuel Arbesman in *The Half Life of Facts*,[3] who suggests: "Facts—whether about our surroundings, the current state of knowledge, or even ourselves—provide us with a sense of control and a sense of comfort…when facts change, we lose a little bit of this control." Aha! Can it be as simple as realizing that we believe that if we can identify, quantify and categorize, we are controlling our universe?

I find it interesting that, as I review the people who shout loudest about the need for more and better research, I often seem to observe this pattern of reductionist thinking in people who are less interested in doing their own soul-searching physical and emotional work. Those more interested in working on their process through the safety of "evidence" call for more evidence. If we're in the business of creating safety in self and others, and I believe we are, then it seems to me that those who seek their safety exclusively in science are missing out on intuitive safety. That safety is more powerful than the scientifically manufactured kind.

In *Blink*, Malcolm Gladwell[4] tells us in various ways that too much information actually causes us to make poorer decisions! One research project demonstrated that when subjects were overwhelmed with too much information to process, they made less favorable choices than when they discounted the information and went with their gut instinct. So, though science may be important, overreliance on information gathering, scientific research and reductionist thinking can be detrimental.

I'm bolstered by some important figures in the human growth movement who weigh in on the intuitive side. Hay and Schulz's recent book *All is Well*[5] endeavors, successfully I think, to marry logic and intuition. For all the affirmations Hay has created over the years for specific metaphysical causations and healings, Schulz has found documented scientific research that supports each of Hay's claims. One of my favorite early quotes: "Just like needing both tires inflated on a bicycle, you need to balance emotions and intuition with logic and fact. Both extreme logic without intuition and intuition without logic breed disaster. We must use both of these tools to create health." I believe intuition is scorned by those who trust only science, to our collective detriment. I'm as interested in results as anyone, but I don't believe reductionist, rational thinking is the only tire of the bicycle that needs to be inflated.

And while it could be argued that Hay and Schulz have simply found the "stories" that agree with their worldview (don't we all?), they're supported by far earlier thinkers (though Hay's been on board for many years), such as physician and missionary to Africa, Albert Schweitzer: "Medicine is not only a science, but also the art of letting our own individuality interact with the individuality of the patient."[6] And here is one of my favorite quotes from Dr. Sarno's TMS model: "There is a woeful trend toward 'body parts medicine' that fails to see people as individuals. A patient is simply a collection of body parts to many of today's specialists. Patients receive a diagnostic label and receive treatment according to an 'evidence-based model.'"[7]

One may perceive me as being anti-science…that's not the case. I'm not suggesting that intuition is always reliable or that science isn't valid. I'm impressed and awed by research with stem cells, with internal bacteria that cause weight gain or loss, with space exploration, with new stories and discoveries being developed every day: it's amazing to me what science does and what it gives us. If I as an intuitive thinker can appreciate science, can scientific thinkers appreciate intuition?

I'm encouraged by some of the science that's now coming forward: a recent article by Bordoni and Zanier[8] talks to the anatomic connections of the diaphragm and the influence of respiration on the body systems. In this paper, in addition to detailing anatomically what the diaphragm muscle is and how it connects to the rest of the body by muscle, nerve and fascia, a major conclusion seems to be the continuity of the tissues through the bodymindcore. There are those in medicine and science who appreciate the spirit of the body! Their concluding quote: "The patient is never a symptom localized, but a system that adapts to a corporeal dysfunction… In presenting this review, we hope to have made a small contribution towards perceiving the patient as a whole and to have spurred new thinking." Welcome words!

Science *or* intuition? Perhaps this dichotomy is best analyzed by Thomas Moore: "Medicine today appears to fit snugly in the age of science. We treat the body as an object unrelated to emotion and meaning and spiritual power. We deal with organs and body parts as separate entities unrelated to the whole. We not only train doctors in science; we enculturate them, make them see the body as an object, and require them to honor the scientific method and be wary of any alternatives. We measure advances in medicine largely by the sophistication of the machines we introduce into a hospital and by new research in pharmacology. In our doctors we admire professionalism, competence, and objectivity."[9] In other words, we send them out on a one-wheeled bicycle.

Since 1927 when Heisenberg introduced his uncertainty principle, we've known that the observer of the experiment becomes a participant.[10] As soon as one puts energy to an experiment, the outcome is shifted. I see this as true for healing... When we hope and expect patrons to improve, our thoughts and feelings begin to convey that change and allow them to find a new pathway. Can we accept the truth that by and large, whatever, whomever (and however) we touch, we affect? And that every individual will respond to every touch in every situation differently?

If part of a healing relationship is about what a client or patron feels comfortable receiving, up to and including placebo treatment, why shouldn't we allow them to seek treatment from a totally intuitive "healer" with no training or credential whatsoever? If they get better from what we might see as a "sham" treatment, are they less better? Even if their relief is only temporary, doesn't temporary relief rekindle hope? Is science, with its possession of specific facts about and control over a situation, superior to intuition, with its ability to receive inner guidance that enables one to act from an unscientific, inner knowing in any situation? Should people be forced to accept scientific authority when they personally trust intuitive guidance? And shouldn't we be working to foster every individual's intuitive guidance *as well as* offering them the science behind our work? It seems that scientific thinkers can become "stuck" in their own heads, and intuitive feelers get "stuck" in their guts. Both miss the full picture.

Douglas Nelson, in *The Mystery of Pain*,[11] cites research showing that among the variables which help people get better is the practitioner partner's ability to present the possibilities in a positive light: "The presentation by the provider as to the value of the intervention is extremely important to the success of the therapy. Research has shown that if the physician emphasizes the side-effects and low probabilities of a particular medicine, the effectiveness rate suffers... In the end, the best approach seems to be to acknowledge the power of belief and to carefully use it for good."

Let's look at placebo as a piece of the healing puzzle that science has used too often as a weapon against alternative therapies. Sugar pills may be effective in helping people feel better, scientists argue; but no real healing is occurring if science can't prove it. These scientists will therefore assume the pain or condition will return, and it may do so. Yet, couldn't it be argued that if someone feels better after a treatment, it doesn't matter if the treatment is placebo, or even "sham"? Shouldn't we care less about the how and why and celebrate the result, even if it is temporary? Why should science get in the way of someone's feeling better?

Interesting recent research on placebo effect comes from Ted Kaptchuk at Harvard Medical School.[12] He's been experimenting with giving placebos to patients for years, but since 2010 he's taken his research to a new level by explaining to patients, before they receive the placebo, that there's absolutely nothing medicinal in their drug or treatment. The amazing result he's finding is that even when people *know* they're receiving a placebo, *if they're feeling cared about, they feel better*—almost as much as when they're receiving placebo without knowing it. Much of the time neither of these types of "treatments" are that far behind standard conventional medical intervention in pain management, and satisfaction results.[13] Most interesting: The placebo effect seems to be "dose-dependent," such that "the more care people got—even if it was fake—the better they tended to fare." Clearly, we have a lot to learn about how easily we let science invade and control a space where it just may not be effective in the absence of its often more caring partner, intuition.

This also brings us to the "nocebo" effect, in which any stimulus, treatment or intervention a person feels is harmful to them, actually is. Research by Paul Enck, Fabrizio Benedetti and Manfred Schedlowski has shown how something perceived as being harmful to the body, a "nocebo" ("I shall harm," instead of "I shall please"), actually will make people feel worse.[14] "What we "placebo neuroscientists…have learned [is] that therapeutic rituals move a lot of molecules in the patient's brain, and these molecules are the very same as those activated by the drugs we give in routine clinical practice. In other words, rituals and drugs use the very same biochemical pathways to influence the patient's brain."[15] So ritual and caring follow the same pathway as the best drugs we have at our disposal. Why, then, do we not pay more attention to the healing potentials of "ritual," intuitive care and the creation of safety, rather than simply prescribing an "evidence-based" procedure or medication?

Gil Hedley is creator of a dissection video series that studies the material most anatomists throw away—the connective tissues that give shape to the human form. Hedley seems to also look for the soul of being instead of the dissection of the various layers. In his book *The Heart of Service*,[16] Hedley suggests: "In fact, quite a few different sorts of problems manifest when a person learns a bunch of stuff like this at a head level, without connecting to it more deeply from an emotional place as well, or integrating it even physically… Doctors who fall into the error of believing that the body is nothing more than a fancy machine can be found treating their patients more like cars than persons. You don't need to talk to a car to fix it, after all."

I often return to Oschman's lecture about science as "stories." I'm as guilty as the next person of selecting those bits of evidence that support my ideas: research "stories" I agree with, I quote as good studies, while those that make less sense to me I sometimes discard or ignore as possibly flawed. It's the nature of us all to judge: I hope I'm discerning instead.

Whether scientist or intuitive, I believe we're all chasing safety. Can we agree that whether we seek our safety through scientific control of our universe, or through the intuitive guidance of a deeper/ higher power, when we land on only one side of this dichotomy we constrain and limit safety in our patrons, therefore constraining and limiting their healing?

So I suppose I'm asking those with scientific minds not to let go of their need for science and knowledge, but to suspend their negative judgment of intuition and consciousness. Our scientific community hasn't even always figured out how to create the true research questions, much less observe and record results correctly. Trying to control all variables is probably impossible. Witness Kaptchuk's placebo research: we're only getting close to the correct questions when we back off, take a breath and realize that science, in its desire to analyze, label and control our Universe, makes progress when it remembers to also think outside the box.

CHAPTER 4

WHICH MODEL OF HEALING?

ANY MODEL!

The great mistake—one that infects world politics as well as the family of therapies—has been when we take what is fascinating to us, the aspects of reality to which we are present, as the real, normative, or ideal, and dismiss other dimensions as illusion.

Don Hanlon Johnson[1]

...the movement of slowed down or static energy of one sort or another is seen as a major goal of much healing work attempted.

Noah Karrasch

There's an old joke that any practitioner of any discipline will do their best to identify any client's sickness in terms of their own model: A nutritionist can "heal" you with the proper foods and supplements; an orthopedic surgeon can heal the same problem by giving you a hip replacement. A colon therapist will clean out your plumbing; a reiki practitioner will move universal energy through your body. A psychotherapist will goad your psychological issues to the fore and help you resolve or release them; a bodyworker or chiropractor will straighten out the kinks in your spine and connective tissues. A surgeon will cut out the offending part; a general practitioner will give you a short consultation and a pill. A hypnotherapist will talk to the subconscious holding patterns. A physical or movement therapist will teach you how to use your body more effectively. All these tools are valid; yet, obviously, none works in every situation. And all rely on two things: the participation and belief of the patron in the technique and practitioner, and the restoration of the free flow of

GETTING BETTER AT GETTING PEOPLE BETTER

energy through the bodymindcore. I've often thought a great slogan for any clinic would be "We move stuck energy."

Most models of healing focus on one specific locus of the body: The psychotherapist/counselor or the hypnotherapist works with the head, perhaps the heart and sometimes the groin as well; the bodyworker, movement therapist, physical or physiotherapist, though working with the entire body, primarily evokes the core or gut to release head, heart or groin. The nutritionist or colon therapist devotes energy to the cleansing and freeing of the gut; the sex therapist strives to free the groin and its issues (which may reside in the head). I don't disparage any model of healing work, just as I'm fairly sure no model fits every person's needs. Some of us will do better with direct bodywork; some want to talk through our issues. Some thrive on nutritional work and others gain ground with movement therapies. There is no "one size fits all" in the work of getting people better.

I believe all good therapists of any discipline combine science and intuition to evoke and connect the head/heart and gut/groin of their patrons. Any therapy model might be served by seeing its method's particular theories in terms of a larger picture which understands the need to move energy through all four of these major energetic and emotional centers. We'll return to this idea in Chapter 8. This chapter is not a comprehensive list of techniques; I'm interested in presenting a survey of techniques and looking for commonalities.

Oriental medicine and the chakra system models have understood this simple energy movement principle for centuries. Acupuncture and acupressure are based on the idea of moving energy up and down the body through meridians. Most practitioners stimulate a particular stuck spot on a meridian, either by direct pressure/stimulation, or by stimulation above or below the stuck spot. Chakras are seen to be too closed or too open; these systems rely on balancing the energies up and down the line so that energy flow is consistent. Many healing modalities owe at least some degree of effectiveness to this respect for the free energetic flow through the body. My own CORE® Fascial Release work specifies the need for a head/heart/gut/groin model of alignment and energetic flow.

John and Eva Pierrakos created a model of healing called *CORE Energetics*,[2] based in part on the work of Wilhelm Reich and the refinement of that work by Pierrakos and fellow Reichian student and disciple Alexander Lowen, in Bioenergetics. In my interpretation of the CORE Energetics model, Pierrakos saw the person as a three-layered being: The *core*, or center of right energy, is the essence or the place where a person lives, perhaps the consciousness or being. I'm beginning to think of this core place as being physically located in the psoas muscle, which carries and anchors the vagus nerve, my "nerve of well-being." The *body*, or second layer, has protected, and perhaps still protects, the core being from the third layer, its *environment*. Pierrakos' model of health invites the client to release holdings in the body to free the core so it can interact with the environment. His wife Eva's contribution in *The Pathwork of Self Transformation*[3] was simply stated: Feel and process your feelings instead of censoring and storing them. All their work centered on recognizing and fostering that free flow of energy through the body and into and out of the environment.

This work was inspired by Reich's orgasmic or orgone energy work. Reich believed that some type of energy, which he named orgasmic energy, got stuck in the body, contributing to dis-ease. He had great success curing many illnesses, including cancer, in the 1940s and 1950s by means of a machine he called an orgone accumulator. Unfortunately, the term "orgasmic energy" raised hackles on some; he was censored, put in jail, and his healing machinery, misrepresented by a disciple, was confiscated and destroyed. The free flow of energy couldn't be allowed if the word "orgasm" was attached. A head and heart were learning to work with a groin, but too many heads objected to their groins being awakened. Though Reich's work closely mirrored much of oriental medicine's "sexual kung fu" with its belief in the need to move orgasmic energy through the body, his ideas were too radical for the Western mind.

Pierrakos and Alexander Lowen, two of Reich's main disciples, created the work of Bioenergetics, which preceded CORE Energetics. Their addition to Reich's work was the concept of the body developing "armor" to protect the status quo; they refined psychotherapeutic bodywork that encouraged the resolution of this body armor.

Pierrakos, Lowen and Reich seem to be echoed by Jack Painter in *Deep Bodywork and Personal Development*: "When we are really alive, the core and shell disintegrate; our energy moves easily from outside to inside and from inside to outside. There is a balance between the larger extrinsic muscles, which give power to our movements, and the inner intrinsic muscles, which give subtle direction and stability."[4]

Peter Levine credits the work of Reich as being key to his development as a therapist. In his model of trauma release, specifically with PTSD, he works to keep clients in their bodily sensations as opposed to allowing them to explore feelings exclusively: "…feelings accessed through body awareness, rather than emotional release, bring us the kind of lasting change that we so desire… Trauma [that] represents a profound compression of 'survival' energy, energy that has not been able to complete its meaningful course of action… If we can gradually access and reintegrate this energy into our nervous system and psychic structures, then the survival response embedded within trauma can also catalyze authentic spiritual transformation."[5]

In the TMS model, Sarno suggests that many if not most of us begin our illness with psychosomatic influence. Our emotions indeed affect the way we feel, much more than most of us have realized. He contends we're addicted either to perfectionism or "goodism," based on our own self-esteem issues, and that we've created or allowed our pain so as to keep our feelings repressed. We're deluded into believing we must manage the world—perfectly. "In my experience, the state of anxiety, which is perceived by the individual as a psychological malaise, is a *reaction to what is being repressed*, created by the ego as a distraction, much as it creates depression and physical pain for the same purpose."[6]

Berceli's Trauma Release Process involves the realization that trauma or stress makes us go fetal; the flexor muscles on the front of the spine (psoas/diaphragm/iliacus) contract and cause the extensor muscles on the back of the spine to tighten and shorten as they are inhibited in response. This condition is known as "flexor withdrawal."[7] Berceli's exercises are designed to lead clients into a shaking sensation as these tightly held muscles begin to release the tension and trauma they've retained and reused any time a new stimulus comes at them.

By releasing the original trauma, Berceli believes we can resolve the current as well as the past difficulty.

I trained many years ago in the Ida Rolf Method of Structural Integration®, also called Rolfing. A biochemist and scientist, Dr. Rolf believed that gravity was the therapist; when gravity got flowing appropriately through the body, then spontaneously the body healed itself. She worked to release the fascia or connective tissue layers of the body which caused the kinks, shortenings and tightening in the body. Though she wasn't thinking specifically about the release of energy, she was moving stuck energy with her work. And though she shied away from the emotional release that often happened during sessions of her work ("All this metaphysics is fine, but make sure you've got some physics under it!"[8]), I believe that Rolfers with their bodywork were working toward goals similar to those of practitioners who work with emotions—the release of stuck energy.

I've modified and adapted Rolf's philosophy and technique into my CORE® Fascial Release work, and still find that the only dis-ease is slowed-down energy. It was Rolf's intention, and mine, to find the stuck spots, introduce them to the client, and ask the client to get bigger than the past trauma being stored as information that is still held in the tissues. This release of trauma restores the movement of energy through the tissues and the body.

Dr. Rolf credited Andrew Taylor Still, founder of osteopathy, with the discovery of the importance of fascial resilience (note that term "resilience," with reference to Levine) in a healthy body. Old-fashioned osteopathy, as practiced more fully in Europe (and in some locales returning to the US), involves connective tissue releases in the body very similarly to Structural Integration. Chiropractic work focuses on creating space between spinal segments to allow this same energy flow. All these techniques focus on touching something on or in the body to create release throughout.

Recently I met Dr. Jo Steenkamp from Pretoria, South Africa. His SHIP (Spontaneous Healing Intrapersonal Process) model of psychotherapy likewise looks at the slowdown of energy, in his case in the mental realm. Like Dr. Rolf, he's interested in creating a space for change, then triggering his client to look at the stuck material, stay with that stuck place, and decide to get bigger and resolve the issues. I'm surprised and pleased at how similar Dr. Steenkamp's work in the psychological realm is to my own in the physical realm. He asks the client to acknowledge the feelings in the body, stay with the feelings and sensations, and decide to overcome them and release/ resolve them. Like Dr. Rolf, he pokes on the stuck spots, using words more often than physical cues. I'm reminded of wise words from his book: "At the very centre of our being we have the need to be loved unconditionally by the people we call our parents, and it is this love that we keep on searching for in adult life."[9] In Steenkamp's model, the free flow of energy is often based on dislodging the traumas we acquired in early life that still make us feel unsafe, unloved or unlovable.

I suspect Steenkamp would support Sarno's idea that we become ill because of the emotional component or the psychosomatic damage to our bodies…what Sarno calls the Tension Myositis Syndrome. Like Steenkamp, he suggests we revisit and acknowledge trauma in order to release old information. And like Levine in *Waking the Tiger*, previously mentioned, all understand the power of the mind in releasing the trauma of the body by seeing it as body *and* mind—or even, as I like to call it, bodymindcore.

A hypnotherapist, like a psychotherapist, is interested in changing mental patterns; they simply suggest that many people can do so more effectively if a censoring part of their brain shuts down to let a deeper area take charge to change habits quickly.

All of the techniques I have mentioned are enhanced when the caregiver works to improve communication skills.

In addition to the bodywork modalities mentioned above, other therapies also feature movement and in some cases movement awareness, which in some ways bypasses the head in favor of gut and groin: out of the head and into the belly. A physical therapist will usually try to teach a patient either a new way to create motion with a specific muscle whose energy has slowed, or how to find and strengthen other muscles around it to take on some of the functions of that tired, damaged or paralyzed muscle. Teachers of Alexander Technique, Feldenkrais work, Pilates and other movement therapies also try to help their clients find the most appropriate core line from which to move, work and live. Yoga, Tai Chi, Aikido and other movement and stretching arts call for flexibility in the body and mind to create that energetic flow we all crave. I'm reminded of Pete Egoscue, author of *Pain Free* and many other books, whose basic premise is that all ill health is based on what he calls "motion starvation."[10]

Nutritionists, colon therapists and practitioners of visceral manipulation (which seeks to identify and release stuck energies through the stomach cavity) are all clearly most interested in releasing stuck gut energy. Whether by moving energy through introduction of herbs, through more thorough evacuation of the colon and a "scrubbing" of the colon's walls, or simply trying to restore function to the organs residing in and around the gut by means of palpation and release, the flow of energy is paramount.

Sex therapy, something we tend to shy away from discussing, encourages the free yet appropriate flow of sexual energy through the sexual organs and lower body, as well as through the entire system. As in Reich's system described above, the idea of creating a flow of orgasmic or orgone energy and realizing that it doesn't need to be stuck in the groin and only occasionally released can certainly stimulate the flow of energy everywhere.

The Body Electric School of therapy focuses primarily on restoring the flow of sexual energy and making the connection between eroticism and spirituality. It was originally developed to restore male sexual energy, but on visiting their website recently I found separate trainings dedicated to the movement of sexual energy and sexuality through female as well as male bodies. Both genders are invited to explore their sexuality as spontaneity, and to stop censoring sexual feelings without examining them.[11]

Energy healers (Reiki practitioners, aura readers, Barbara Brennan students and others) seek to restore energetic flow wherever the body suggests it needs help. Spiritual and faith healers simply ask for divine guidance and intervention, try to create that sacred space and invite healing to flow into any affected area of the client/patron.

Undoubtedly I've omitted some therapies and in so doing disappointed their practitioners. That wasn't my intention. It's impossible to mention every type of therapy in this chapter. The thesis I want to propose is this: as distinct from more traditional allopathic or scientific medicine, *the movement of slowed down or static energy of one sort or another is, or needs to be, seen as a major goal of healing work*. The technique can be as simple as asking God to heal a body by bringing in Holy Spirit or other religious or cultural energy. The technique can be as esoteric as trying to create an energy flow in the head (brain and nervous system), heart (heart and circulatory system), gut (stomach, pancreas, liver, spleen and digestive system), or groin (bladder, sex and reproductive system). The technique can mix with other models: the physically based connective tissue, spinal system, musculoskeletal system, digestive system, lymphatic system, nervous system, or emotion-based therapies can all be effective in this energetic restoration. Many effective caregivers see the goal of a session as the creation of more energy flowing through more of the the body more easily. Can we encourage our doctors to consider this model? As Thomas Moore says, "This is the time for us all to become healers of persons rather than technicians of the body."[12]

In *The Multi-Orgasmic Man*, Chia and Abrams talk to the universality of this energy across cultures.[13] "The idea of chi is not unique to China. Dr. John Mann and Larry Short, authors of *The Body of Light*, count forty-nine cultures around the world that have a word for chi; the words vary from *prana* in Sanskrit to *neyatoneyah* in Lakota Sioux to *num*, which means 'boiling point,' in the language of the Kalahari !Kung." We may have different words, but most of us understand that there is an energetic flow, or a lack thereof.

And let's open the next avenue…eventually we'll talk to the use of groin in this healing partnership: If energetic challenge is happening, whose groin is involved, what's appropriate, and what's unethical? We'll examine all manner of combinations of practitioner head/ heart/gut/groin centers working with patron head/heart/gut/groin centers in pages to come. We'll think about how to work with the energy of each of these centers in both helper and other. We'll talk about how to prevent the crossing of ethical lines.

I have no more business being a preacher or teacher of ethics than any of us; I've had my shortcomings and failures in ethical behaviors.

I have tried to use them as learning experiences and hoped that I haven't damaged patrons in learning my many lessons. I don't think anyone expects any of us to be perfect all the time, or to make the correct moves in every situation. I think we are expected to continue to self-correct, so that our mistakes are both less severe and less damaging to self and others. I think this self-correction needs to be never far from consciousness, particularly when another person has entrusted their core to our help. Our respective professional ethical codes notwithstanding, we will all make mistakes, but we must not lose sight of the fact we're ethical when we're considering the rights and opinions of our "other."

From this viewpoint, I'm reminded of Kylea Taylor's premise in *The Ethics of Caring*: "Ethics is the process by which we sort out what best creates inner and outer harmony in our lives… What I do affects you. What you do affects me. What I do to you will ultimately affect me… The degree of our willingness to delve into the dark truth of our own motivations, desires, and fears will determine our ability to be caring, flexible, and ethical… Ethical behavior is reverence for life demonstrated by right relationship to another."[14] No matter which helping model we use, can we agree on Taylor's ethical advice?

Some years ago I attended a day-long seminar on ethics based on Jungian archetypes. Sunny Cooper[15] from the Pacific Northwest brought this idea to the Midwest. I found her concept intriguing and thought-provoking: "Archetypes are patterns of energetic influence which manifest in humans as behavior patterns, roles, interactions with others, and as our life challenges. Archetypes come into our lives as guides and teachers of the important lessons of our lives." I see archetypes as patterns or models of personalities. Many of us choose to assume one or more in a desire to form our most effective personality. Basically Cooper paired several archetypes together and suggested that ethically, we should be aware of our need to create the kind of client that matches our archetypal framework and choices. She listed four types of "healer" categories: magician, rescuer, nurturer and sage. She then paired these categories with archetypal client categories: magician attracts destroyer; rescuer finds victims; nurturer finds children, and sage attracts seekers.

Cooper's point is that if we're not operating carefully and ethically, we'll tend to attract to ourselves mostly those people who fit our category and seek our particular style of validation. A magician will attract destroyers so they can help them rebuild. If we're a rescuer, we'll often attract victims who need to be rescued, and a nurturer will attract "children" who need constant nurturing. If we see ourselves as a sage, we'll primarily attract people seeking to receive wisdom from us. Cooper believes that ethically we serve the public better when we create our own balance by understanding our archetypal stance and remembering to let it serve as guideline rather than guiding light. She believes it's unethical to let the practitioner self get "stuck" serving only one narrow and limiting/limited population.

This possibly unconsious selection of the "perfect" seeker for our type of help can apply regardless of the healing modality we practice, and we'll revisit it in Chapters 9 to 12. Pierrakos in *CORE Energetics*[16] and Brennan in *Hands of Light*[17] also talk to the idea that whichever form of mental illness we as practitioners, or as patrons, carry will often make us seek someone of a sympathetic pattern: for example, a psychopathic personality, who could be seen as a persecutor, might seek oral personalities who will become their victim(s). Such an oral type practitioner, focused on gratification through the mouth, might thus either ingest or suck in too much of the psychopath's process, becoming their victim. They describe this connection in terms of energetic "hooks" or "streamers." Whether we're allowing transference or countertransference, we still are operating from our own egos. It makes sense: we all seek those who can fill our needs. Are we as therapists still doing this?

Likewise, if we see every patron or client who comes through our door *only* in terms of the model of healthcare we deliver, we're probably abusing some of those clients. Nutrition, while important to anyone's health, may not cure that sore shoulder more quickly or better than bodywork, which in turn will not necessarily address irritable bowel syndrome (though both techniques might surprise us and remedy these respective problems). Just as we don't want to attract only the people who fit our archetypal construct, we also don't want to retain clients who could be better served by others.

P.N. Forni (see *Choosing Civility*[18]) gave a sound bite definition of civility in a lecture I attended: "benevolent regard for others." I believe too many of us get into the habit of believing we're supposed to "fix" someone else…either by becoming their master/magician, their warrior/rescuer, their parent/nurturer or their teacher/sage. Doesn't "benevolent regard" suggest that what we really want to give those people is tolerance and non-judgment, which will feel to them like empowerment? Can we understand that our role is to *not* assume the mantle of authority for them and their process, but to communicate to them how they can find their own authority? This key invites us to maintain that benevolent distance of non-judgment as we foster their resilience.

An article by Lael Katharine Keen which crossed my desk challenges us as practitioner partners to get better at listening to the boundaries our clients, patrons and patients set for us: "To be ethical, every time we go to touch some one we must remember that all our skill can take us no further than the doorway of the client's world, where we must stop and knock and wait for the invitation to come in."[19] I like the concept that we should remember we are truly empowered only when our patrons invite us into their bodymindcores.

I've long been wary of people who believe they have answers for others: I remember a quote about being suspicious of proselytizing men, and being suspicious of *me* also… I continue to feel that anyone who preaches to me that they have my answers is stealing my power, my health and my choices. This is not ethical; this is rape. This, I believe, is why, years ago, a client pointed out to me that the word "therapist," broken down, spelled "the rapist."

So, what is one's intention when approaching patients, or patrons, or clients? Whatever our technique, are we still operating in the model of tricking, rescuing, parenting or teaching, thereby stimulating fight, flee or freeze? Or in our model are we knocking at the door, then coaxing and enhancing that which is already in the client to open, express, feel, blossom and move forward?

To summarize this chapter, I use a quote from Mary Sykes Wylie in *Ethics of Caring*: "Blind allegiance to a particular therapeutic model becomes an ethical failing when the therapist consistently gives more weight to the model than to what clients say they want and need."[20]

What are the across-the-board traits that nearly all effective healers share to some degree? Let's revisit Jerome and Julia Franks' book *Persuasion and Healing* to see their conclusions. We'll look at the four main characteristics they have found to constitute effective healing, and contrast them with other models to see where the commonalities lie.

CHAPTER 5

WHAT GETS PEOPLE BETTER?

*…intractable fear prevents a person from
returning to balance and normal life.*
Peter Levine[1]

*When we feel heard and externally validated without
judgment, we feel safe. When we feel safe we're better able to
take risks. When we take risks we have a greater chance of
making changes. When we make changes, we can heal.*
Noah Karrasch

How do we help to re-morale-ize clients? How do we help them
restore their resilience and banish their aloneness and anxiety? Let's
follow more fully the four steps the Franks set out as commonalities
of successful healers in *Persuasion and Healing*: caring, creating safety,
communicating, and cooperating. Let's see how all four of these steps
could be seen to be based on Porges' wisdom that helping people feel
safe is paramount. Toward the end of this chapter we'll visit other
models that offer support for the Franks' findings.

STEP 1: CARING

Do we really care about our patrons?

Basically, most of us didn't go into therapeutic work for wealth,
though some probably had that goal, and may have achieved it. But
given the cost of most training courses and the years involved in
credentialing, money was probably not the only, or even the primary,
consideration for many of us. We got into the work because we
cared about people and wanted to see them well and happy. People

can feel this caring, or lack of it. They know when a practitioner would rather be somewhere else. I remember a student who years ago confided he was always happier to see a patron leave his space than to see them come in the door. Why bother to expect business with this attitude? He went from eight patrons in his first week of practice to three in the second week. I'm not sure if there was a third week in that practice.

While the allopathic model of limited communication and caring is changing, some medical schools still try to remove much of caring from their doctors-to-be, because they believe it's not a good idea to get attached to patients. I'm glad to say this old model seems to be disappearing as we realize that the simple act of caring makes people feel better just because they feel cared for and about. I return to *Healers on Healing*, where Rollo May says, "In my view, the fundamental element of all healing is empathy. The word empathy sounds like sympathy, but its meaning is actually quite different. In the present context, it means that the healer does not promote healing in the patient by commiseration or sentimental feeling, but by a kind of subtle communication. In empathy there is a nonverbal interchange of mood, belief, and attitude between doctor and patient, therapist and client, or any two people who have a significant relationship. Empathy is the experience of understanding that takes place between two human beings."[2]

Thanks to my early teacher, psychologist and rolfer Stacey Mills, I've long accepted the difference between sympathy and empathy. Stacey suggested that when someone is stuck in a well, sympathy causes one to jump in with them; ultimately no one is helped by this action. Empathy is demonstrated by throwing the sufferer a rope. Can we remember to hold this distinction, and not allow self to get caught up in the sympathy game? As Jo Steenkamp says in his practice, "Empathy is the stimulant for healing; sympathy is its killer."[3] Are we investing in our clients by empowering them, or are we enabling them in their patterns?

I've also recently become intrigued with the word "empath," a word most of us use to describe someone who quite easily absorbs thoughts and feelings of and from another. If we adopt this word, we could also define a word possibly coined by me: of "sympath," which denotes to me someone who *absorbs too much* from their patron or partner. As most strong empaths know, there is a challenge in not letting oneself become the sympath in a relationship. As Stacey Mills always told us, "Don't go jumping in that well!"

So empathy might be compared favorably with caring. And while caring about another externally validates them, this boost from without can trigger an internal validation which can restore or introduce resilience in a seeker who feels non-judging safety from an empathic partner. When we learn to listen to our patrons, offer when invited, be with them without judgment, and explain how we might help, we create a space for their stuck energy to return to its desired movement. Caring looks and feels like trying to truly know them, their concerns and goals. Caring looks and feels like helping them to discern these goals they can't yet find. Caring is non-judgment when another shares their burden of guilt, shame or grief. Feeling care from another gives patrons permission to admit they're confused, tired or in pain; and helps them see that while they may claim some responsibility for their condition, they don't have to fault themselves for it.

I'm reminded of a video I recently viewed called *Healing Neen: Trauma and Recovery.*[4] The video told the story of a young African-American woman who had experienced a trauma-filled life including homelessness, drug addiction and prostitution. She found her way to a much more productive world and dedicated her life to helping others resolve their trauma. One quote made me realize how much she cared for others. She told a group of female prisoners: "Everything that happened to you, happened to you. You didn't do it to yourself." Yet too many of us feel the need to assume the blame for the trauma, the too much information, that's happened in our past.

When we feel heard and externally validated without judgment, we feel safe. When we feel safe, we're better able to take risks. When we take risks, we have a greater chance of making changes. When we make changes, we can heal. I remember a description by Scott Peck of a client's process toward healing in his book *People of the Lie*[5] "...[she] gradually came to realize that, unlike her mother, I had a consistent and genuine respect for her identity and the unique individuality of her soul." Can we give that respect to each seeker? He also speaks of the "atmosphere of acceptance" which the practitioner must create so the patron can feel respected and safe; then the real work can begin.

Berceli describes this "atmosphere of acceptance" thus: "The difficult part of this process is that only we can explore this inner place of pain, anguish, and craziness. We must go there alone. However, it's important to be tethered to a lifeline held by a close friend, therapist, or guide. Going into this place without an objective observer can cause us to get lost in the internal chaos. Having someone who holds the other end of the line of reality facilitates our return to the realm of sanity."[6] **Can we care enough to hold this line for our patrons?**

Stan and Christina Grof wrote a book describing her "spiritual emergency."[7] When Ms. Grof realized she was mentally and physically unstable and unable to deal with her personal process, she confessed to her husband her fear that she was going crazy and that if she let herself go, she couldn't find her way back. He offered to hold her hand through the process, and they were both astonished to find themselves in a three-year process to bring her back to health. I see this story as a true example of caring for another, and a depth to which I'm not sure most of us could commit as the healing partner.

Moore, again: "Patients have an inborn, essential pride. They don't need or want to be humiliated, and there is every opportunity in medicine to humiliate… Since illness and the medical culture already put people in a humble place of suffering and passivity, they need an added measure of assurance and positive recognition."[8]

I recently began working with a new patron who told me fairly early in her first session that she needed to be in control of how much change was going to happen in her life. I reassured her that it was ultimately her decision how much to change, or even whether to change, or whether she could and should retreat further back into her box. That had to be her decision, her choice. At the end of her final session in our series, I suggested she might want to experiment with allowing her heart to be the first part of her body to arrive in any situation. Her response, which I thought was brilliant: "I'll not do that, but I'll begin to let myself think about it."

For me this represents an example of coaxing the patron and allowing them to decide just how far they're willing to move in a new direction. We're all unqualified to push people faster than they're ready to go; none of us is ready for that task. Levine has spoken to this problem effectively: "At the same time, too rapid or large a magnitude of expression can be frightening, causing a client to contract precipitously against the expansion."[9] He invites us again to realize that if we truly care about others, we'll let them unwind at their speed instead of our own.

I remember a discussion I attended years ago which featured a world-famous doctor on a panel. An audience participant asked the question: "If a doctor feels there's no hope for a patient, ethically, should he continue to treat?" I thought it was an excellent question! The doctor, however, simply laughed and said, "Well, if that were the case, I wouldn't have many patients." That told me so much more about the doctor than I wanted to hear! If we have no hope and can find no hope for a patron, how are we possibly serving them unless we honestly confess our lack of hope and admit we can give only palliative care? If we can't care enough to believe when they need someone to believe in them, or at least sit with them as they examine what they can't yet find their way through, can't we care enough about them to send them down the road so someone better equipped can have a chance to help?

By contrast, too many practitioners, especially of massage and counselor variety, sometimes care too much and end up trying to live another's life for them. They call to "check up" on patrons frequently, they give extra long sessions when they feel progress is being made, or especially when they don't. They move the boundaries for their special people. A middle ground suggests we learn how to care for others, and let them know we care, while maintaining a professional relationship. Our goal is to help others stand alone; not on top of us.

As an aside: I tend to find etymology intriguing. Remember my liking for Steenkamp's E-block or emotional block; I also think of E-motion as Energy in Motion. So I find it interesting that evil is "live" spelled backwards, and the devil is "lived" backwards. When I look at the words "well" and "ill," I notice that *I* am in "ill," but *we* are in "well." And hell may truly be as simple as giving our personal power, our "ill" or "well" away to a third party "He." "He" can't fix you; you've got to get up and get it yourself as you relate to that other and create that "we."

Years ago, a patron shared how several different therapists had told her it was time to get over her grief…her mother and grandmother had been dead over a year, and it was time to move on. In the larger context, her mother and grandmother were her only friends; her father and brothers simply took advantage of her and added nothing to her life. When she lost her two best friends in the space of a year, she was demoralized. She needed to grieve satisfyingly and needed help finding the way to do so. No one seemed to care enough to help her; their best response was "It's time to get over that." I suggested to her that the time to get over your grief is when you get over it, and no sooner. With this simple permission, this space to grieve without feeling judged, she began to get better.

We all understand that some people are hard to care for! I used to be thankful I adhered to the Ida Rolf ten-session model of therapy: When I was uncomfortable with a client (the role I assigned them in those days) for whatever reason, I knew that I probably wouldn't see them after ten sessions. Very often an interesting thing happened, however. As the series of work progressed and I got to know and empathize with the client and their pain, I found myself understanding their hurts more clearly, and often times liking, if not at least being able to tolerate them more fully. My initial judgments were tempered as I began to allow myself to understand their thought processes and their journey. I don't think anyone wakes up and says to him- or herself "I'm going to be the worst person I can be today."

When we walk that mile in someone else's shoes, we begin to realize they didn't set out to be an angry, unhappy, ungenerous or demoralized person; they've merely responded to life the best they could and created the best self-validating system they could make. *We've each become the person our chosen responses to life's events created.* As I learned to understand others and worked to comprehend their motivations and behaviors, I found myself better able to care about them. And as I became less judgmental, I found they became freer to self-discern, self-disclose and drop the mechanisms that were holding them back. They became able to feel that internal validation as I validated them from the outside.

But what if you truly can't stand a seeker? What if you dread their arrival? What if you want them out of your life? This is tricky; it's neither caring nor therapeutic to "fire" a patron, yet there are times when you're reasonably sure you're not the right partner for their therapeutic relationship. The first question for self as healing mirror/ partner is: "What do *I* contribute to this situation and why?" It may be as simple as realizing the patron reminds you of your mother, or childhood babysitter, or ex-partner. It may take some time to identify the behavior or trait that triggers in you the unfavorable reaction. It's worth your time, their time and the time of your future patrons for you to try to deal with your resistance to the other.

I return here to Levine: "Consider the alignment to that of shamanic traditions, where the healer and the sufferer join together to re-experience the terror while calling on cosmic forces to release the grip of the demons. The shaman is always first initiated, via a profound encounter with his own helplessness and feeling of being shattered, prior to assuming the mantle of healer. Such preparation might suggest a model whereby contemporary therapists must first recognize and engage with their own traumas and emotional wounds."[10] Levine suggests to me that if we're *truly* caring, we'll have done our work first, so that our patrons and their processes won't be soiled by our judgments.

I remember the old test for deciding when to speak: "Is it kind? Is it true? Is it necessary?" There are times when I suggest, as lovingly as possible, to someone that I don't think I'm their appropriate practitioner. I usually suggest we try three sessions together; if neither of us feels progress is being made, I try to steer them to someone else who I think may be more helpful. Even if I do feel progress is being made after three sessions, I don't want to hold them to me if they don't feel that change. If they choose to acknowledge the difficulties we seem to be having making progress and decide they want to stay and explore that difficulty, I'll stay and work with them.

Sometimes I'm surprised when someone tells me how much good they feel they're getting from our work, when I'm seeing neither release of problems nor resolution of them. Other times they agree with my suggestion that we don't seem to be creating a team; they don't want to invest more time and money into that goal, and decide to seek help elsewhere. I feel better for having made the offer and having put responsibility for their health choices back with them. And they usually respect my integrity more fully as they realize I both assess the situation to sense the poor fit, and give *them* the control of their situation and their process. I want them to succeed! I want them to feel cared for, even if I'm suggesting they go elsewhere. I try to care enough about my patrons, and about myself, to pursue only relationships where I think I can be of help to them and myself. My desire to care for and create safety for others often keeps them returning until they feel safe enough to release and resolve trauma and move forward on their own.

I'll return to my earlier mention of my career as a musician, and add to it the brief span of time I spent trying to be a salesman. As a musician, I realized that when I truly cared about my patrons and wanted them to experience a good evening out where they were part of the show, we all had a great time and the tip jar was full. If I was focused on making money, somehow patrons could sense this and stayed away! Likewise, when my partner was selling crafts at local shows, we found if we hovered over the booth and critically eyed each potential customer, they quickly moved on...yet if we made ourselves available somewhere in the distance, we could easily tell if they were interested in her wares and wanted help. We had more successful sales *and* enjoyed the shows where we relaxed and absorbed the atmosphere of the craft show, the other crafters and the patrons. In both cases, when I truly cared about the "other" and their experience, my own experience was enhanced. Can we transfer this truth to our sessions with patrons in this career?

Thomas Moore sums up caring: "...ultimately it is the soul that heals... When you treat people as objects, as cases and syndromes and machines in need of repair, you will not be a healer, not even a doctor or nurse. You will be a technician, a human repairman, a functionary in a world of objects. Soul will not enter into your work, not into your skillful use of techniques and not into your relationship with your patients. Your work will not satisfy you, not because it isn't worthy work but because there is no soul to give it a deep human pulse."[11] I don't believe we can define the art of caring better than by suggesting that *soul* must be present to allow another to feel safe enough to face their fears and move through them, holding our hand.

To summarize this section on caring I'll again cite previously mentioned placebo researcher Ted Kaptchuk: "Genuine healing is a journey, facilitated by a healer, into a broken and hurt self, the purpose of which is to encounter a depth of humanity deeper than the tragedy of any illness. The healer takes a person into the disorder and brokenness, whether it is curable or incurable, to find an intactness and reconciliation that profoundly reflects and manifests the genuine self."[12] If we can't care about our patrons, how can we lead them on this journey?

STEP 2: CREATING SAFETY

Is it safe to breathe?

I once had a session with a practitioner about whom I'd heard great things. I knew she was working from someone's house, as she lived out of town. On arriving at her "office" I found myself standing on a rickety front step of a derelict house in a marginal area of town and ushered through a filthy entry hall into a cluttered and dirty room that smelled of too many cats on a very hot day. After being told to strip to underwear and lie on her table, with no sheet under and no drape above, I received what was probably a very good treatment. I couldn't tell, because I couldn't get past the smell, the clutter, the unhygienic table, the music she preferred, my modesty and the stifling heat of the room. I didn't feel safe or cared for and I didn't feel that setting lent itself to my being healed. I did see that practitioner again, but never in that setting.

It's simple, really: most people feel safer and more comfortable in a beautiful, orderly and harmonious setting. It's not hard, or shouldn't be hard, to keep such a setting. An office that feels something like a factory, where the patron sits in a large waiting room with gray walls, old magazines, noisy children, complaining receptionists and staff who flit from area to area without any acknowledgment or kindness, isn't conducive to feeling cared for. And an office that has a negative tension hanging in the air because its occupants don't work well together doesn't encourage one to release feelings or fears or truly examine blocks or expectations. Most of us hold our breath in such a setting.

On the other hand, some people won't resonate with a different practitioner's concept of safety: a darkened room with candles, incense, crystals and New Age music doesn't please everyone! Some people expect sterile, some crave cozy. Can we span the gap and offer both? The setting we create will dictate the kind of seekers we attract. If we want the New Age crowd, an esoteric setting may be just fine. If we want people who are serious about making changes, the charts and art on the wall, the furniture, the colors, the harmony of our space need to reflect our desire to create comfort as well as knowledge as we coax their innate ability to release and resolve trauma. Most practitioners want to instill healthy breathing in patrons and clients; are we providing what makes *them* relax, or what would make us relax?

Sometimes setting has nothing to do with the physical space itself, but the way the practitioner creates the space with their words and expressions. A horrible learning occurred for me years ago, when I was relatively fresh to this work. A new female client was standing before me in her underwear, clearly uncomfortable at being that vulnerable and a bit nervous about being visible from outside, even though the windows of the room were high enough that there was no chance of this happening. As I observed her in the style I'd been taught, I said, "Now, let's see a couple of big breaths." I couldn't understand why this woman absolutely crumpled in front of me; then, as I reviewed my words, I realized she thought I had asked to see a couple of big *breasts*! Though she managed to have the treatment, she never returned for a second session. I realized the power of my words, the power of communicating both positively and negatively. This experience made me ever more careful about which words I chose to use. It was also a catalyst for my giving patrons the option to remain fully clothed during our work, as I began to understand safety in that instant.

I've noticed over the years that people who don't enjoy having their feet touched (and in fact react strongly and run away or seem to check out of their bodies) have often (not always!) been abused sexually in their childhood. I've found when someone can't stand this touch, I've got to slow down and make them feel safe again; coax them into their feet, talk in a reassuring manner, tell them exactly what I plan to touch and why, and keep them present in their body while I work. No playing dead! It makes sense that someone who was touched inappropriately on the lower half of their body would try to run away, shrink their energies up towards the head and brain, and choose not to be touched on the lower extremities. It's often a strong clue as to what's happened in the past. Most body talk is a clear and vital cue, if we learn to look and listen.

I was recently shown a chart created by Finnish researchers, in which study participants were asked to document where in the body they felt particular emotional currents, or thought those sensations lived.[13] Their resulting drawings from several different cultures were quite similar, enough so that the researchers felt the study was significant. I found it interesting that only happiness produced a sensation of warmth and energy in the legs; anger and love also mildly registered a positive energy or grounding there. Sadness, shame, anxiety, depression and envy showed a tiny bit of cooler energy in legs. Other emotional states produced energy in the upper body, but there was little energy registered below the waist in most emotional states. This suggests to me that, for the most part, we truly do suck our energies up towards our head and away from groundedness and a desire to live in this our human condition. We feel unsafe on the planet and respond throughout our bodies.

Possibly the most moving assessment of the creation of setting comes from Rachel Naomi Remen, who suggests, "I've discovered that basically I don't know what's needed. But if I listen to the client, to the essential self of the other person—the soul, if you like—I find that at the deepest level of the unconscious mind, the client knows what's needed. If I can be present at that moment, without having any expectations of what the client is supposed to do, how he or she is supposed to change in order to be 'better,' what happens is magical."[14] Remen demonstrates to me her understanding of the creation of a safe and non-judging setting for her patrons.

To some people the physical space isn't even important when they feel this emotional connection and trust with the practitioner; this soul of relationship and relationship of soul. They're willing to "e-mote"—to put their emotions back into motion.

STEP 3: COMMUNICATING

Do we explain what's happening, and why?

Years ago when I first began working in England with individual clients, I thought I'd better brush up on both my English and my communication skills. Therefore I developed a fairly standard talk for meeting each new patron and explaining to them clearly what I thought my model provided and how it worked. I was gratified that perhaps 85 percent of the time, on hearing this talk, they would respond, "That makes sense." To me, a great part of the session's work was already done if I received this response. I realized that if the model made sense to seekers, we were well on the way to moving their energy and resolving their trauma.

I teach many continuing education and professional development courses, as well as my own model of bodywork to massage therapists. I'm continually amazed how many healing partners lack basic communication skills. I often challenge students to talk to their patrons: telling them what they're doing, why they're doing it, how it may help, and what the patron can do to assist in the process. It's intriguing how tongue-tied some practitioners become when faced with this challenge.

I'm only half joking when I suggest I've become a cheerleader for my patrons during sessions: "Good, now we're into a spot that needs to release...take a deep breath, stretch that left leg and right arm. Great, keep your back down, and take a long, slow breath...that's it! That's right where you want to be...can you feel that change? Did you feel a release? What are you feeling right now?" There are even times when I'll verbalize for them the fear or pain I sense they're experiencing when I touch a particularly sensitive area. That way, they know I know how scary or painful the situation has become. I find the better I communicate what I want to help them accomplish in a session, the more they understand that goal. Then, the more they know I know how difficult it is for them to stay with the process, the better we can accomplish our goals.

Dennis Chernin in *Spiritual Aspects of the Healing Arts* describes this process in this way: "The role of the holistic physician includes open and effective communication with patients. He demystifies medical care by explaining both theory and treatment. Also he stresses individualized treatment, which requires that he know each patient individually."[15] Schwartz in *Healers on Healing* says it thus: "...therapists need to become educators. People must be given back the power to take charge of their own well-being—a power that is often taken away from them by systems of health care that tend to create dependence...the healer becomes more like a mapmaker or guide..."[16]

As I mentioned earlier, I have several "sound bites" that I can use to explain what I'm doing and why. I may rely on charts, pictures, a skeleton, or tracing lines over a client's body to explain to them where we're going and why. The more I can make them see their bodymindcore in my model, the better my chances of getting them on board for the changes I can see them making to release and resolve the old, stuck trauma's effects.

And a large part of communication is listening! It's amazing to me how many practitioners do a quick intake and decide to get to work. As a bodyworker, I still look at people as they come in and make a quick assessment before I look at their short intake form's information. However, the best single tool for getting to know what we want to do in our time together is to ask, "So, what's going on in your body?" before getting out of the way and listening! As I mentioned this phrase in a recent class, one student said, "I just say, 'What's going on for you today?' That takes it out of the body realm and allows them to tell me anything and everything that might be helpful." Too many of us seem to believe we're supposed to be the expert and so should discern what the patron needs. If we'll give ourselves more time to listen, often we'll know exactly what's needed. Often patrons try to give their power to me: "What do you see? What's wrong with me?"

Though I'll give them my evaluation, I still want their feedback. They live in there—what better authority could I find?

Sarno shares how he spends a great deal of time in his intake asking questions about his patient's childhood and their current personalities, in addition to asking about symptoms and pains: "Of primary importance to me is each patient's psychosocial history…with particular reference to the personalities of parents and relationships with them;…to list stressors in their lives…"[17]

Often I suggest to people their intake form contains the major pieces of a jigsaw puzzle, and I hope they'll put down all the pieces they can think of. I liken this jigsaw puzzle to a picture of a goldfish that might turn into a bowl of oranges, if we can only find the correct piece to show us the entire picture. This metaphor seems to encourage them to search through their memory bank to retrieve earlier assaults to the bodymindcore that may have some relevance to the current condition. Quite often as we work, more pieces of the puzzle come to light that didn't make the intake form. We recreate health, piece by piece.

Rita Charron in *Narrative Medicine: Honoring the Stories of Illness* suggests: "Doctors, nurses, and social workers practice in new ways today as compared to their routines of even a few years ago…the notion that doctors and therapists bear witness to patients' suffering is beginning to be heard and considered…eight-minute visits do not suffice to expose all that must be said…"[18] The current medical system may want to change, and with enough aware practitioners on board, perhaps we'll overcome the attitudes that make an eight-minute visit be termed a consultation.

As a bodyworker I'm continually amazed at the number of patrons who have been through a medical model and treatment, yet felt totally unheard and invalidated by the treatment from and relationship with their doctor. Too many people, including me, have had poor communication experiences. During my largest health crisis, that plane crash in 1987 that debilitated me, caused me to have spinal surgery with fusion and Harrington rods, my partner (a professor of communication!) and I spent time writing down the questions we had for my doctor's daily (and expensive) visits. We were tremendously disappointed that on each visit he was already backing out of the room on question two. We never received satisfaction from this doctor. Eventually I fired him.

While I realize our current US medical model (bottom line, profit; what else?) dictates that the doctor spend a limited amount of time per patient, that very model has lost sight of the fact that *each person has a story that needs to be heard and unwound if they're to get better*. Often, simply listening to a patron's concerns, even if our response is only "I don't know," makes them feel heard, validated and reassured. Admitting our own fallibility empowers our patrons. I've had many people tell me how much they appreciate a practitioner who isn't afraid to admit they don't have a perfect answer as they consult and listen. Listening only costs a bit of time, and frankly, I believe it's far more cost-effective than the current medical model that's being practiced in too many allopathic factory systems.

I'd be interested to see the results of a research project where doctors give one half of their allotted time with each patient to listening to the patient unwind and convey their symptoms and fears, and only talk or respond when answering those concerns or asking for more information or clarification. What if the first half of the allotted time was for listening and the second half for making suggestions?

As caregivers, we could enhance our communication skills by learning to be better reflective listeners. If we truly want to be empathic with our patrons, we'll want to develop better listening skills. Reflective listening suggests to me that when a patron tells us about their condition, fears, pains or feelings, we respond by restating what we think we've heard and inviting either an agreement that this client feels heard, or a corrective restating from them so we better understand what's going on for them. Too many of us don't bother to wait and really try to hear what someone has to say, and absolutely don't bother to stop, reformulate in our own words what we think we've heard, then ask them if we're hearing them correctly. How demoralizing! True and careful restatement of what we think we've heard is a skill too many of us don't possess, and don't strive to possess. Listening denotes empathy; empathy denotes caring. Do we care enough to communicate with effective listening?

Gladwell talks to this problem in *Blink*: "Patients file lawsuits because they've been harmed by shoddy medical care and *something else* happens to them. What is that something else? It's how they were treated, on a personal level, by their doctor."[19] Patients who feel heard, listened to, respected and valued don't sue their doctors, even when results aren't good. If and when they feel part of the decision-making process every step of the way, their ownership allows them to take responsibility for that process. Gladwell finds these "good doctors" who don't get sued have three things in common. First, they're more likely to make "orienting" comments, explaining a bit of who they are, what they offer, how they plan to work as a team. (They explain their model.) Second, they're more likely to engage in active listening to their patients. (They create a safe setting.) Third, they're more likely to laugh and be funny. (They care.) Isn't it intriguing that these simple communication steps, some of which have nearly been bred out of the medical curriculum, are so important to the patient/patron feeling a part of the healing team?

Even more intriguing to me: Doctors who aren't afraid to apologize for their mistakes, face to face with patients and their families, have far fewer legal complications and malpractice issues than doctors who adhere to the idea that Doctor is God, and therefore makes no mistakes.[20] When we as practitioners admit to our humanity, we put ourselves on an equal footing with our patients/clients/patrons. Referring to the earlier placebo study: Even when one knows placebo is given, one feels better for the relationship created. When people feel cared for, respected and safe, they feel better. Relationship is important! People want to share humanity with their medical team. The medical world has tried to take that option away, but seems to be returning to a more human and humane face.

Moore supports this idea: "You don't have to have any special goals. You just listen and talk…present yourself as a professional and be a human being… A first step…is to receive what a person has to say. Let the patient set the agenda…The second step is to encourage talk…"[21]

I return to Sarno because he has so many good thoughts: "Another crucial therapeutic element became clear early on as well: the person must not only *understand* the nature of the process but be able to fully *accept* it as well. Not faith, but acceptance of the idea is essential."[22]

If you can explain to a patron why you believe they're currently unwell, and if they can accept your reasoning, they can get better. And could it be that the ability to hear and process such information is yet another definition of resilience, which Levine tells us is the key to resolving trauma?

So, I find that the more I can allow my patrons to be their own authority, telling me what's going on in their body and world, what's their fear, their pain, their anger, the more I know about how to serve them. If I can get them to realize their pain or disease is the summation of their stressors, I bring them on board. If I then explain to them what my model of work is about and how it might help them, and get them to agree to try my model as a participant, we're often going to get them better. Our communication can make them feel cared for, safe, not judged, but valued and heard…all validations from the external world, that trigger the ability to self-validate and find health.

STEP 4: COOPERATING

Do we do to them, for them, or with them?

We've already briefly considered Step 4: What is the patron's part in this work? Too many people, especially of an older generation, still expect their doctor or practitioner to "fix" them and their problem. Many people would rather have a knee replacement than learn to do a few simple stretches and exercises each morning that might realign the problem spot in their knee through the hip and foot, taking pressure off the painful area. Many people would rather have surgery covered by their insurance or subsidized by their government than seek bodywork, physical therapy or chiropractic treatment that asks them to work to change habits so as to enhance or restore their own energetic flow. Many think if insurance doesn't cover a procedure or technique, it must not be valid. Many people want to find a counselor to just listen, or better yet a psychiatrist who can give them a magic medication to take away their anxiety, instead of trying to understand the source of that anxiety and deal with it. People have to participate if they're truly going to get better!

Jack Schwartz says this well: "…one aspect of the healer's love is to help the client overcome the fear of change…technique is actually just a form in which the therapist's unconditional love can be transferred… But we must make it clear to people that they also have to start recognizing their own needs."[23]

And Berceli gives us a good clue in terms of getting the work from the patron instead of delivering it to them: "I have worked with many trauma survivors in my career as a therapist. This experience has taught me that, at a certain point in the recovery process, each person goes through a phase that requires some kind of reinventing of themselves."[24] If we can't get someone to participate, take some responsibility for their process, and choose a different way of being, are we going to get them to make any real changes for the better?

I recall wisdom from Patricia Norris, in *Healers on Healing*: "The therapist's role is to teach the patient to heal, to be both coach and cheerleader in this process…"[25] I really resonate with this image. It seems to me that Steps 3 and 4 are honored as we get better at communicating to others what we're trying to do and how it will be helpful; then asking for, directing, encouraging and praising them for the deep work we're coaxing from them. We foster their resilience. In *The Ethics of Caring*, Taylor suggests that a practitioner's main job is more that of a midwife than a strategist: "the therapist permits, protects, and ushers forth that which wants to happen of its own accord."[26]

So we are practitioner, healer, helper, caregiver, healing mirror, healing partner, therapist, educator, mapmaker, assisting guide, cheerleader, usher, emotional midwife, provider. These words and concepts begin to define the model in which the "authority" removes some of the societal or medically imposed expectation of taking responsibility for another's health and returns it to the patron, who ultimately could and should be the authority for their own health process. People who wish to be patients instead of patrons will often see you as a different type of figure, as Thomas Moore says: "…as saviors, magicians, confessors, geniuses, and even lovers… Don't get caught in the fantasies by playing the role."[27] Or, as Douglas Nelson says, "One of the substantial benefits of the partnership approach to the doctor–patient relationship is the sense of control it gives the patient, and that sense of control lessens the experience of pain."[28]

When I'm working to cheerlead and encourage my patrons, I often not only ask them to do a bit of work in the session, but also usually give one or two ideas at the end of a session to enhance what we've just done. I hesitate to use the word "assignment" as some people will work too hard to accomplish an assignment. A movement or awareness cue that I suggest they "play with" can often truly ice the cake of what we've done in a session. It may be as simple as drinking more water or breathing more deeply and often. It could be motivating them to remember to walk around the block daily, or to sit straighter at their computer as they raise the screen and lower the keyboard. I might suggest they say the thing they need to say to the person who's most irritating them, or write down the grievances they still hold against their parent, child, significant other, or some other nemesis. I might ask them to consider working with a counselor to resolve that which comes up and out of them. I challenge them to find a way of letting energy flow more fully through their bodymindcore. I encourage them to take the work from the session out into their world. I don't give three ideas; one or two is sufficient. Three can be overwhelming so that none gets remembered or practiced.

This world has become such a fast-food world: everyone wants instant results. Health doesn't work that way. While there are occasional spontaneous healings, and while some people may seem to resolve long-standing issues in an hour's time, most of us have to dig in and do some work. Since many seekers don't yet understand this guiding principle of true healing, it's up to the practitioner to inspire them towards doing their own work, with guidance.

Here, then, is the core belief I take from Frank and Frank: Success in therapies comes from caring, creating safety, communicating and cooperating with patrons to make changes. And in this instant-gratification world, most of us don't have time or energy to seek safety; we've lost our resilience. We tighten our core lines and tiptoe through the eggshells or hot coals of life. We as healing partner practitioners can do more to help these patrons and clients feel safe in their world and on this planet, simply by recognizing lack of safety as the beginning of health challenges and following these four steps to help patrons feel safe.

Author Stanley Krippner[29] suggests that the healing stool has three, not four, legs. First, certain personal qualities of the practitioner appear to facilitate the client's recovery. Second, the client is expectant and hopeful that feelings of healing can occur. Third, the client chooses to create and/or accept a sense of mastery. Again, caring and safety begin the process. Hope only rises when safety and trust are present.

It's interesting to me how, if one looks, one finds clues to healing in a rather disparate set of readings. I'm thinking now specifically of *Teaching with Love and Logic* by Jim Fay and David Funk. While describing how to become more effective teachers, they identify four components to a process; when these four steps are dealt with, teaching and learning are enhanced. Their steps are: 1) Identify the problem. 2) Identify whose problem it is. 3) Show empathy. 4) Offer a positive relationship message. This simple distillation of the message of their book shows true similarity with the models of healing featured throughout this one. A last message from Fay and Funk: "No behavior technique will have a lasting, positive result if it is not delivered with compassion, empathy, or understanding."[30] Again, and yet again: Do we care about our patrons? Do we tend to their safety and self-esteem?

Elizabeth Kübler-Ross suggests that her four pillars of healing are trust, faith, love and humility. In so many ways, each of these authorities is using slightly different words to define the same attitudes that effective "healers" bring to their patrons.[31]

Levine[32] suggests a nine-point formula that provides support and potential healing for clients. Note how most of these (although there are more of them) fit into the Franks' model (as indicated within square brackets).

1. Establish an environment of relative safety. [2. Create safety.]

2. Support initial exploration and acceptance of sensation. [3. Communication.]

3. Establish "pendulation"* and containment: the innate power of rhythm. [3. Don't push too fast, but leave the client in charge.]

4. Use titration. [3. Communication/monitor how much the patron can accept.]

5. Provide corrective experience by supplanting the passive responses of collapse and helplessness with active, empowered defensive responses. [4. Participation.]

6. Separate or "uncouple" the conditioned association of fear and helplessness from the (normally time-limited but now maladaptive) biological immobility response. [3 and 4.]

7. Resolve hyperarousal states by gently guiding the "discharge." [2 and 3.]

8. Engage self-regulation to restore "dynamic equilibrium" and relaxed alertness. [4.]

9. Orient to the here and now, contact the environment and reestablish the capacity for social engagement. [1, 2, 3 and 4.]

Remembering Porges' model specifying that safety facilitates healing, we can see how Krippner's, Ross's and Levine's models not only dovetail with that model, but overlap that of Frank and Frank: The personal qualities of the practitioner certainly can facilitate recovery. If every patron feels cared for and safe with this practitioner partner, they're probably more ready to accept healing and less defensive about making change. This feeling of care and safety, combined with this practitioner's ability to communicate their model of work and what may come, what they expect to come, can make a seeker expectant and hopeful. Someone who feels safe and cared for understands what is being done to try to create change, and as a willing participant in that change process chooses at least to consider creating and/or accepting mastery over their condition or illness or pain.

---

* Pendulation "is about getting unstuck by knowing…that no matter how horrible one is feeling, those feelings can and will change."

CHAPTER 6

RESOLVE OR RELEASE?

...to treat an illness is different from maintaining a state of well-being.
Thomas Moore[1]

Changes don't occur when we allow patrons to rely on us for the release they want instead of challenge them to the resolution they crave.
Noah Karrasch

I was recently given a thought-provoking article written by Carmen Littlejohn[2] for a Thai massage audience, inviting therapists to consider the difference between *releasing* a stuck muscle and *resolving* the underlying physical or emotional issue that allows the muscle to stay stuck. What may seem like a small distinction between the two words actually illustrates very well the problem many practitioners seem to have when they allow themselves to touch symptoms instead of core issues. For whichever of many reasons, some of us mainly work to release that built-up pressure of another's issues instead of trying to find out how to actually take away the problem. In other words, shall we be satisfied with simply releasing the stuck energy, or should our goal be the resolution of the physical, mental or emotional issue so that energy continues to flow freely? It's a worthy task to try to resolve; but is it always possible, or even ever possible? Clearly, relief is more common than cure...which are we seeking?

Recently in a conversation with a colleague, I described how I've come to feel that too much of what passes for therapy, this resolve *or* release, could be termed "buying a support network." Years ago, I thought a therapist I knew was unethical because I heard she'd been treating the same client weekly for years and years. I didn't share my judgment with her client's partner who was telling me of this arrangement, who next said, "Yes, he doesn't like attending alcoholics meetings, so he pays her for a private meeting." I still don't personally approve of this kind of therapy, and I don't think I'd either seek it or provide it. But if it's all a client is ready for, release instead of resolution, then that's what one must give them…or send them on down the road to someone who can feel satisfied providing release work.

Rolf talked about "core and sleeve" a great deal (if core is the deepest layers and our essence, then sleeve is the superficial, external and extrinsic of the body); Pierrakos describes the center of right energy as "the core." Reich talked of the "core orgasmic energy," and Steenkamp strives to reach "the core issue." Listen to Steenkamp's words: "The moment you *make* people feel good by means of an external source, you have distracted them from the internal healing process. Facilitate the internal healing or the connectedness, and the outside balance will follow suit."[3]

Many of us as practitioners claim interest in getting to the core issue: how many of us truly give energy to the belief that core issues can and should be resolved, and therefore establish resolution as a treatment goal? And how many of us are instead satisfied with the temporary release, a pressure-cooker petcock bleeding off of core issue energy? Ted Kaptchuk puts this well: "The healer takes a person into the disorder and brokenness, whether it is curable or incurable, to find an intactness and reconciliation that profoundly reflects and manifests the genuine self."[4] Clearly, release is on the way to resolution, but resolution of brokenness is a far more exciting and satisfying destination than release of symptoms.

On reading Littlejohn's article I was totally arrested by the pairing of the two words. I'd been severely challenged by an advanced student who comes from a different discipline, and realized I often slip over the line into release work. I'm not discounting its importance. Yet to me, consistent release without the intention to resolve is frankly just another pill or palliative. I hope people will realize they can make changes and then make them. Changes don't occur when we allow others to rely on us for the release they want, instead of challenging them to the resolution they crave.

For years I've likened some people's use of therapy visits to the act of cleaning their clothes closet. Too many patrons take everything out of the closet; all or most of the emotional issues, the dysfunctional relationships and challenges they've suffered (though most of us leave a couple of unexamined boxes deep in the back…). They look at each piece of clothing (each issue, problem, relationship, pain) but decide they've got to keep this shirt/feeling because Aunt Helen gave it to them; they've got to keep this pair of pants/behavior pattern because they may lose weight again; they've got to keep this hat/ habit because it reminds them of a fun time, they've got to keep this pain because it's become their identity, or because letting go of the physical pain might let them feel their emotional pain. They can always find a rationalization, a *"because"* that allows them to put that shirt or that behavior pattern back in the closet. In the end, they put every piece of clothing/each behavior back into the closet, or bodymindcore, even though they've realized they'll probably never use many of the pieces they've just saved.

What have they released? Precious little! They've only tidied those feelings of disorder and that mild to serious internal churning of their self. They've straightened the hangers and put things back in a more orderly fashion. What brokenness and disorder have they resolved? Yes, what *have* they resolved? Too much therapy seems to allow this type of soft cleaning instead of an honest and effective tough-love scouring. Too many people seem to believe they're accomplishing change if they sit with a problem for the specified amount of time, then put its atoms back together and get on with life in the exact same frame.

Are we challenging for change, or simply allowing symptom release? I agree with Porges that we seem to be anchored in fight, flee, or freeze too much of the time. The fourth figure on my adrenal dial reads "feel." I've described previously how I can see some people hiding, freezing, running away from my work. Having recognized this behavior, I'm getting better at keeping them in their bodies. If someone wants to leave their body while I change the oil, it just won't work.

There's an old country song whose chorus line is about your heart being in it, and not wanting to be intimate with a body whose heart isn't in it… The "it" becomes a multi-dimensional word. Your heart's not in the body? …in the relationship? …in the process? …in the moment? How can change occur, beyond a mild release? How can we find resolution if our heart's not in it?

I've mentioned Gil Hedley,[5] the fantastic spiritual anatomist who points out the continuity of the body's tissues and the patterns of trauma stored in them. In his videos one clearly sees how different bodymindcores store tension and trauma in different places and ways. Some of us store extra tissue around our stomach or back or thighs or heart. Eventually the extra tissue becomes glued to the next layer of tissue; a type of paralysis results, the energy slows down, and we end up developing dis-ease in the physical place where energy has slowed or stopped moving entirely. We're motion starved. It's a bit like the closet metaphor above; we forgot to air out our closet, release the unnecessary, rotate the stock and keep all in good working order. One can barely release if one won't move energy; it's even more difficult to resolve this stuck-ness.

In my bodywork sessions and classes, I talk to patrons and students about layers one, two and three. I believe the layering model actually transcends bodywork and can be applied in any of the "healing" modalities. Layer one is actually fun, relaxing, restful; it's nurturing without challenge: a release in a gentle massage, a drink to unwind and vent with friends, a beauty therapy session, a superficial chat with a therapist about the week's activities. Layer two is the spot where the patron is present and participating, and feels challenged but nurtured through deep bodywork or other intense therapy. Seekers may not be certain they want to stay on this layer, but when they do stay with it, and release, they hopefully begin to resolve.

Layer three is the overdose—too deep, too fast. Patrons feel attacked at that center of right energy and so shut down, check out, dissociate, freeze, play dead, become demoralized or run away; in some way deciding to leave the process to the facilitator and their own vacant shell. Their core has flown, frozen, or occasionally fought. At all cost, however, they seem to believe they must *not* feel.

The practitioner partner has overachieved and the patron partner is overwhelmed. We've over-triggered them. Are we getting release with such a person? Maybe we are—Ida Rolf seemed to push her clients extremely hard and had success. Are we getting a resolution? That's less certain.

Levine talks of "too deep, too fast" work: "Frontal confrontation is generally ill advised: to 'attack' resistance directly is likely to intensify it or to break it down precipitously. Such a sudden demolition of a defense is likely to bring with it overwhelm, chaos and possible retraumatization."[6] He affirms for me the idea that damage is done when we keep people poised on that deep layer three, instead of nurturing their exploration of layer two as it approaches layer three.

A worthy goal with our patrons, then, may be to take them to the top edge of layer two and keep them present without pushing them into that layer three shutdown, and at the same time keeping them focused on both their feelings and their body. Most practitioners and researchers I've mentioned in this book would probably agree that good work is done only when we keep people actively engaged in the dissolution of their old patterns instead of allowing them to disengage or freeze. Certainly this is echoed in the Franks' steps three and four, in which we explain the model of treatment and the patron's expected participation in that model.

Let's discuss one more interesting concept: the idea that we as practitioner partners can take on the "stuff," the negative energy, the pain, the psychic difficulties, the unresolved thought forms of our patrons. In our desire to be empathic we can become what I earlier called a "sympath." A sympath lets empathy overwhelm them to the point where they suffer and endure the bodymindcore pains of (and for) others instead of helping them resolve such pains. The patron may temporarily or even permanently feel much resolution after such a session, but the practitioner partner may feel totally altered, and actually devastated after such a treatment. What do we do about this problem? Some of us absolutely could be identified as the highest paid housekeepers in town; vacuuming rooms, cleaning closets, straightening disorders and returning next Tuesday to do the whole thing over again. How can we practitioners keep ourselves from becoming a housekeeper who merely picks up after this immature other, instead of teaching them to keep their own house in order? How do we keep from feeling more and more worn out by, and resentful of, their irresponsibility?

To me the *empath* is able to understand the feelings another person is feeling and have a pretty good sense of what's going on for them, because they easily put themselves into another's shoes, or bodies or minds. This is a talent, and I think a worthwhile one. It allows us, foremost, to show others we care about them and understand them—our step one. Empathy lets them feel less judgment coming from us when we're able to say, and mean, "I think I know how you feel." But why feel what they feel *and* allow ourselves to get bogged down in their feelings? Why take on their pain, their anxiety, their grief or shame or fear? Why become the sympath? Why jump in the well with them?

Can we learn to understand and empathize with the pain of others without taking their pain upon ourselves, and being the one who ingests a bit of it for them without resolving anything? Can we train ourselves *not* to be part of the support network for sale that too many are seeking? A release for a patron instead of a resolution, with us assuming their pain or grief or shame, is definitely not a resolution for us, either. Unless we, as practitioners, are resolving our own issues, it is unlikely that we will be able to help our patrons resolve theirs, instead of continuing along the route of just releasing them.

Again, Levine: "Many therapists hold to the hope that they can somehow provide their clients with the positive, affirmative (I–thou) relationship that will assuage a client's fractured psyche and restore his or her wounded soul to wholeness. However, what often happens is that a client's dependency upon the therapist escalates and gets entirely out of hand..."[7] I'm reminded of a years-old *Twilight Zone* television episode where a young boy played by Richard Thomas sat by the corpse of his father, the region's "sin-eater." As there was no sin-eater to be found in the area, the son, in a fit of grief, began eating the food from his father's corpse, thereby ingesting all the father's sins so the father could move on to the next world sinless; but also adding the sins of the father to the son's own collection of sins. This of course meant he'd inherited the sins of generations, to his mother's chagrin. I've often thought some therapists *want* to be "sin-eaters" for their patrons. Perhaps this is why so many "helping" professions understand the need for continued supervision of practitioners, both to keep them from becoming "sin-eaters" and to help them to learn to maintain their boundaries as an enhancement to self-care.

I recently attended an interesting seminar about learning to deal more effectively as therapists with "noxious" people.[8] We as helpers have all had experiences of such people; we as people have all had experiences of such people. I don't believe anyone sets out to be noxious, but I do think many individuals have either physical pain, mental health issues or personality disorders of varying degrees of seriousness that cause them to inhabit an unsafe and therefore painful world. As a result we've chosen to find ways to blame the world for our problems instead of thinking, feeling and working to make changes in our own issues or disorders. I wonder more and more whether simply enabling an ill person to feel safe in their insecure world will help them to abate pain and mental illness, soothe personality disorder, or simply make these easier to tolerate as they learn to love and enjoy their own company and personal universe. But perhaps this step of releasing old patterns will set them on the path toward resolution. Do we point them in that direction? Or do we ingest their difficulties?

A large part of the presenter's advice was common sense; first, taking care of self with diet, exercise and rest. He also discussed creating boundaries that don't allow such patrons to expect absolute healing in the practitioner partner's hands or through their skills. Again, when we expect our patrons to take part in their process, we'll have fewer problems absorbing negative energy than if we choose to be psychic sponges and sympaths.

To close this chapter, I'll return to Will Schutz. His book *The Human Element*, while geared towards creating health in social systems such as workplace groups, rings true for the individual as well: "People must learn why they have not wanted to change, what the payoff is for not changing, and what they fear about the new state. If they are clear about all of that and then decide to change, the program will work."[9] **Resolution** requires honesty; release enables continued hiding.

And perhaps the clearest of all, let's allow Frank and Frank one last thought about the ability or inability to help patrons resolve instead of merely release their challenges: "In terms of this framework the aim of therapy is to make patients aware of their own contribution to the perpetuation of their symptoms and to offer support until they find the courage to take responsibility for their behavior."[10] We can't be the change others desire; we can only be facilitators of that change. If we give sympathy instead of empathy, we'll hurt ourselves while only creating release and selling support instead of resolution. We can offer support, but if we believe we can heal others by ourselves, we'll burn out. Possibly we'll be successful; but we may be unhappy and our patrons may only release symptoms, not resolve wounds. The desire for resolution must come from the patron. Only then can they both release the problem, and resolve it.

CHAPTER 7

PHYSICIAN, HEAL THYSELF

EMBODIMENT

*...the root cause of most physical ailments is connected with
not living in accordance with one's inner guidance.*
Shakti Gawain[1]

*To be a soulful person you have to have made some progress
toward dealing with your own psychological issues.*
Thomas Moore[2]

*Yet, a true practitioner partner strives to invoke cooperation, then
evoke the inner knowing and healing that both of us have within.*
Noah Karrasch

How do we become more effective in coaxing resolution instead of
accepting release? Let's embody... First and foremost we've got to be
practitioners who model for others an honoring of our own process.
This mustn't be a false creation! We can neither pretend we have all
the answers, as too many do, nor live in a bodymindcore that's flawed,
with no acknowledgment of our own humanness. It's all right to be
imperfect as a practitioner; it's not all right to try to cover over our
imperfections and ask others to be something we're not being, or
trying to become, ourselves. Years ago I remember reading about a
"breatharian" who preached to his disciples that one could live on air
and water only. He'd recently been spotted at a fast food restaurant,
stocking up! This is not the embodiment our patrons deserve; "Do as
I say and not as I do" has never been an effective route to resolution.

One of my pet peeves about "helping" professionals runs
throughout this book: I see therapists who seem to be lazy about doing

their own work of taking care of self, keeping self in a bodymindcore healthy state—or, to use an important phrase, embodying health. I believe many of us in the "helping" professions have been helped by someone in a particular brand of healing and so have seen that profession as something we want to attain. This is good. It gives us, as helpers, a sound footing in the "care" category of the Franks' research. Clearly we're so relieved at our release (or resolution if we're really lucky) through the work we've pursued, that we want to spread our good fortune by sharing and practicing this tool that worked for us.

Many counselors have gone into their profession because of their own mixed-up lives. Too many bodyworkers and massagers are crying for satisfying intimate touch, and so give what they seek, or have found bodywork to remove their own aches and pains and want to pass on that relief. Many people in helping/healing professions have landed, or will land, in their field as a result of their own challenges being assuaged through the specific technique they choose to honor by putting their life's work towards it.

Perhaps all these individuals truly believe they've received that deep healing, had their issues resolved and dissolved, and that they're ready to help others achieve their healthy place. Perhaps, one hopes, they have been and they are. Too many of them (us) are fooling ourselves when we believe we've been healed at depth. Too many of us are running from healing in ourselves (beyond occasional release without resolution) when we pursue the process of trying to evoke change from our clients—change we ourselves may still need to make. *Healing is an ongoing process; not a destination to be arrived at, so much as a journey to be enjoyed.* And total resolution may look like ascension—are we ready for that step? Yet, if we aren't working on our own process, chances are we aren't creating true relationship with a patron, and we aren't growing as human beings ourselves.

Occasionally when I evaluate students in my courses, I feel the need to let them know I don't see them embodying the work they want to do. When I use the term "embody," I'm thinking that someone who doesn't work on their process and demonstrate health (taking into account their history) isn't a good representative for their profession. As you can imagine, this doesn't always create good feelings towards me from the student. But if I believe in resolution of stuck energy instead of its temporary release, don't I need to be honest enough to let them know I perceive they're only halfheartedly doing their work on themselves by working on others instead? If a caregiver is unhealthy in their own bodymindcore, should I as a client want to see them professionally? If a counselor is on their fifth life-partner, should I want to trust my emotions around relationships to this person? Should I as an instructor foster that dishonesty, in myself or in them? Sometimes I receive defensiveness from my students for my efforts. Often I'm thanked for the direct and caring evaluation of something they possibly knew in themselves, but hadn't yet chosen to face.

We've probably all heard the term "wounded healer," and usually I subscribe to the idea that those who have been most wounded are in a better position to lead others out of the maze of their own pain. If nothing else, they're often able to demonstrate a resilience their patrons can emulate, and they offer a "you can do this also" model to follow. But a wounded healer can do so much better when they've truly dealt with the resolution of their wounds, instead of accepting the temporary release so many of us crave. Those who simply continue chasing symptom relief in their own bodymindcores are probably going to assist patrons in chasing symptoms instead of seeking true resolution.

Remember my student who dreaded clients' arrival and was glad to see them leave? I encouraged him to seek a different profession, as he had neither physical structure nor emotional ability to work with others in this style, and he knew it! Yet he couldn't resolve the problem. He used substances and people to release his difficulties and tolerate his unhappiness instead. He's me. He's you. He's in all of us.

Emerson is reputed to have said something along this line: "What you are doing speaks so loudly, I cannot hear what you are saying." I remember a massage school student who wore braces on both wrists for carpal tunnel problems throughout her training. She was in constant pain. After graduating from the course, she continued to push herself, hard and fast, through what her face suggested was unbearable pain. Often she'd see eight to ten clients per day for massage, hurting all the while. Though her clients felt her results were usually good, how could she feel good about what she was doing when she was clearly hurting herself with every session? I've always suggested to students that if they are in pain while working, they aren't doing either of the partners in healing any good in that session. Another student was a small woman who worked on athletes for 16 hours a day, until her wrists wouldn't let her work any more. How can we let our actions get so far from our values? As Moore says, "Sometimes the doctor's need to heal is stronger than the patient's need to be healed."[3]

If you're a bodyworker or massage therapist, when was the last time you had a good massage just for yourself? If you're a counselor, when was the last time you saw a professional just to unwind and allow the burdens you've absorbed to be cleansed? How do you take care of yourself? Do you take care of yourself? And do you do such work regularly, with intention; or have you just been following the form without truly staying present? Is your heart in it?

Some of us are good at minding diet, getting exercise and rest, maintaining boundaries and learning to turn off our need to counsel and heal when we get away from our practice. Others of us never let the mechanism stop; we're constantly working to enhance others, and at our own expense. For me, this working on others instead of on self represents a superficial work instead of the core work I think is vital to effective helping of others.

I used to really dislike time alone and would do whatever I could to fill all my waking moments with eating, drinking, socializing and busy work. At some point in time I realized I'd like to work on learning to enjoy solitude. These days, I treasure that time alone and see it as a great part of my recharging. I enjoy being with others and I enjoy my pastimes, but I really enjoy my "do-nothing" time as well. I see it as life-enhancing, which is my definition of good and healthy living. Many of us still try to run away from ourselves, however. We're back to my earlier claim that we expect to be validated externally instead of finding our own internal validation. If and when we can realize that we're enough, we do enough, and we can allow our machinery to achieve neutral once in a while, we offer our patrons a much more effective process to recharge their spirits, and ours.

Do I entrust my process to an emotionally unstable counselor? I've known far too many people who were alcoholics, suffered abusive childhoods, were unhappy in their lifestyle choices, or couldn't sustain healthy relationships, but decided to become counselors after they had received not resolution, but simply respite or relief, release. Is such a person really ready to help others resolve issues if they've simply put a bandaid on their own troubles? I realize we're all in process, and that no one is perfectly reformed or resolved from all their past—very few ascensions can be found in the data. I suggest those who work hardest to "fix" others might want to look deeply into the mirror they're holding up to that other, and more frequently. Only then can they honestly assess whether they're helping others, or releasing their core self at the expense and through the process of others. This thought reminds me of Scott Peck's words in *People of the Lie*,[4] in which he defines evil as imposing one's will on another for the purpose of avoiding one's own spiritual growth.

Another peeve: I've seen business cards from some in healing professions, particularly alternative therapists, which read like a telephone directory: four, six, eight, even ten different techniques that will undoubtedly be able to "heal" you as a "patient." Wow, I try to keep my distance from these jacks- and jills-of-all-trades. The synthesis of so much material into a system that works is a worthy goal; yet somehow these people too often seem not to have synthesized the techniques into a personal style that truly works. Instead, they usually seem to have lots of surface knowledge in their heads but can't see the big picture or major needs of their patrons.

I remember a metaphysical healer I knew who used to brag about being able to dissolve clouds at will, and to manifest a parking place whenever she needed one. I always wondered why she didn't dissolve some of the extra 100 pounds she carried, or manifest a decent car to put into that parking place! Of course we all teach best what we need to learn ourselves, and I again admit and affirm that I certainly have my own work to do as much as anyone else. I don't agree with the behavior of people who pretend to be authorities when their life clearly demonstrates they haven't accepted that they've not yet arrived themselves. I'm reminded that the word "ego" can be seen as an acronym: Edging God Out.

What about any "healer" who smokes, is morbidly overweight, or sustains other unhealthy lifestyle and habits—who doesn't walk their talk? Why would I seek treatment from someone who doesn't demonstrate health and an awareness of it? Why go to someone who gives advice they don't seem to take for themselves? Why go to someone who promises to fix me, and can't give me references of similar cases they've helped/healed? Why visit a practitioner who guarantees my health, but isn't demonstrating their own? Why trust such a person to help me if they "feel" wrong to me? Why not find someone who represents a process of joyful living "on purpose" instead of one who reflects to me what's wrong with the world? Steenkamp says it well: "If someone claims to be a healer who will heal you of your chronic systemic stress reactions, run away. Quickly."[5]

We all know that most idols have feet of clay. In the Bible, God forbids the Israelites, his chosen people, from making idols or graven images, because they aren't representative of the true God. Likewise a "healer" who makes promises to get anyone and everyone better, and therefore encourages dependence on, and even addiction to their techniques and/or personality, is very possibly creating a false idol for their patrons. Such an egotistical practitioner has violated rule number one of the healing code: First, do no harm. By depriving their patrons of self-determination, this practitioner has violated the trust given them by their others.

Jack Painter says this well: "Finding and keeping a new, stable center was essential in my work with others. I could share myself and help others find a new direction, only if I was clear about my own direction."[6] And again, Thomas Moore: "People often talk about the wounded healer, the helper who knows what it's like to be hurt and in need. But there is also the 'healed healer,' the doctor who by witnessing the courage and deep humanity of his patients has become more of a person himself."[7] While doing the best we can as helpers to be the ultimate mirror to each partner who crosses our path, we may sometimes act in a way that seems unfeeling, unhealing, uncaring and unsharing to the partner calling for balance and assistance. It's a delicate balance we try to maintain! Do we truly walk our talk?

Remember, I don't pretend I've arrived…I'm simply stating I don't disguise the fact that I'm in process, hopefully making progress, and that this is what I encourage clients, students and acquaintances to find also. While accepting release, I continually work toward resolution. In my experience, clients resonate with this energy, this striving, this satisfaction with progress while deciding to dig deeper into the process. As I set my intention to do my own work, I attract to me clients who are interested in doing their work as well. They're grateful for my help in guiding their process while respecting that it's theirs, and they're pleased that I'm acting as a partner, not an authority. They appreciate hearing the words "I don't know" from their healing partner instead of a line of rationalization or misinformation or latest theory that may or may not make sense, feel right or begin the resolution process.

And too often, this is a bottom line: Too many of us "helpers" *want* to be an authority because we *need* that boost to our *own* self-esteem, our safety, our purpose for living, our internal validity, our core health. Too many of us want others to respect us, listen to us and defer to our ideas. For me, a true practitioner partner strives to invoke cooperation, then evoke the inner knowing and healing that both of us have within. Every good therapist understands that, like Michelangelo, we're trying to free the statue from the stone; we're trying to free the joyous person from the tangle of issues in which they're frozen. We evoke, we don't change. And we can't make changes in others without admitting we need to remain open to change in coreself. We won't resolve the trauma in others unless we face the trauma in ourselves. We have no business doing the work on others if we believe we need to do "to" them instead of "with" them.

Moore again comes to me as I think on this issue: "A counselor who has confronted herself and doesn't act out her biases and emotional conflicts can help a patient far more effectively than one who simply has learned the techniques… The larger issue is the need of chaplains and counselors to face their own demons and deal with their complexes as part of their preparation."[8]

And to chaplains and counselors let's add bodyworkers, doctors, jacks and jills, and all who believe they're helpers.

If we're honest, and I think most of us want to be honest, I hope we can admit that actually our patrons are there to serve as our teachers. They show us our processes: our frozen spots and fears or fearlessnesses. The relationship can also teach us more about processes in general. We can learn much about a specific disease or a personality disorder as we work with yet another patron. But perhaps even more important is what they teach us in every encounter, about ourselves.

Remember, many or most of us still use the term "practice" as we refer to our work and our business. This has always felt like permission to me—by defining our work as practice, we admit to pursuing learning in each relationship and session. We practice becoming better "others" and better selves-with-others. Depending on our attitude toward our patrons and our work, we either limit ourselves by our need to demonstrate our egoic process, or we humbly grow through every encounter. Where, in balance, do you live and work?

To share or not to share this, our own process, with others? Should we disclose more of who we are and what our process has been, if it seems to be useful to the relationship and the patron's goals? Frank and Frank suggest: "A person's own wounds may enhance the ability to empathize with the sufferings of others. In addition, the healer who has been cured may serve as a model and a source of hope to the sufferer...effectiveness is primarily a quality of the therapist, not of a particular technique."[9] The technique is worthwhile, but the state of the practitioner is even more important. I don't see the Franks suggesting one must share core self over-abundantly, but rather, sufficiently to demonstrate health and healing in a way that draws the client into the process. Jack Painter says it well: "In my work I found that when we as individuals begin to recognize and express our own needs, to find our centers, we want to confront, deeply touch, and share ourselves with others."[10]

What is appropriate to share or disclose about our own process? Some practitioners seem to manage to turn every bit of information a patron divulges into an opportunity to share a bit more about their own process and their imagined achievements in that process.

Others maintain a strict boundary and share absolutely nothing of self. Is there any guiding principle that enables us to judge whether something we might disclose will be helpful to the client? Or should this be left to personal choice on the part of the practitioner, based on their person and personality? How does one decide what's appropriate and therapeutic to disclose? Is there any rule that will serve?

Some practitioner partners are advice-givers—like the counselor, hairdresser, bodyworker, doctor or cabbie who feels the need to straighten out your life for you. Here's what Steenkamp has to say about these "helpers": "Continual advice giving is an indication that the psychotherapist is trying to sort out his or her own problems, not those of the client." And later, in even more incisive words: "It is the observer's own fear of the client's pain that causes him or her to label it as pathology."[11]

Steenkamp clearly sees that any practitioner who plays at making changes is possibly evading their own core changes by focusing on those who come through their doors and "fixing" them. I don't think I can add much to these sentences! I concur with the idea that too many of us practitioners work on our processes through the problems of our patrons. This inappropriate self-work at the expense of the other doesn't really touch and resolve issues of either practitioner or patron. Releasing tension in others while avoiding resolution in ourselves is a disservice, or at least not much service to either. For me, it seems dishonest.

I remember visiting a counselor many years ago at the recommendation of a friend. I gave the practitioner a trial period of perhaps eight or ten sessions. I found at every session her rate of self-disclosure was so high that I felt she should be paying me! I've also been frustrated by other caregivers who didn't offer one word of greeting or encouragement or explanation during treatment. Neither end of the spectrum was satisfying to me. I think we could all aim a bit more for the middle of that spectrum.

I'm suggesting for consideration that all practitioner partners aim a bit more toward a middle ground which takes the emphasis away from "me" (the practitioner partner) and puts a bit more emphasis on "not-me": the patron and their process. If we love to disclose, clam up a bit. If we're a clam, open up so as to let someone know that their experience and pain isn't unique, and that they're not at fault for having it. Where is the middle ground that allows a patron to feel like "us" without losing "me"? I believe if we experiment with our process of reaching toward a moderate position of self-disclosure that allows the other to understand they're not alone, we'll become more tuned to the problems and process they've brought and are grappling to understand, and we'll be of greater assistance to them.

Physician, heal thyself. Realize none of us has yet arrived, or we'd no longer be on the planet. Demonstrate to your patrons/clients/ patients who you are, warts and all. Seeing you be who you are gives them permission to be who they are. Let yourself express your self-validation, your own satisfaction at who you are, your "enoughness," and they'll have permission to self-validate. They'll resonate and receive help. They'll revitalize their own resilience. Bore others with your process and your life's details and they'll run away or play dead. Lecture them on who they should become, and they may try to follow you, but they won't receive the internal validation we strive to uncover—they'll fight or flee. Internal validation will come from their ability to learn and discern from your guidance, not from your taking over their process or forcing them to drink from the fountain of change. This process is about the patron or the other; if you make it about practitioner or self, you're not helping their work.

And yet: All our work is totally about us as well. If we're not honestly evaluating who we are, what we do for self and others, and how it's affecting the greater whole, we're being dishonest. If we can't admit, and celebrate, that we're on the planet to grow as a human being through the healing exchange, we probably should find a different path. Each person who crosses our path, whether as a patron/client/patient, as a friend, or even as a chance encounter at the grocery counter, has much to teach us, if we allow ourselves to be open. Our patrons, our family, our "others" are all our teachers. Are we pretending we're the only teaching authority, or are we still on the planet to learn and grow? Such an excitement for growth defines a good practitioner, I believe.

In the next chapter we begin to examine my model that challenges us all as helpers to consider which parts of our body we operate from—or conversely, where we hide. I ask us to reflect honestly on the truth that where we live, or don't live, in our own bodies, affects our work as practitioner partners. I believe a bit of attention to what sort of self-work remains undone in us will give us an opportunity to do better work with and for our patrons. I'm not suggesting we *must* change behaviors to become better; rather, that we all allow ourselves to be vulnerable to our own flaws so as to evolve into even more effective healing partners. Warning: These coming chapters are a work in progress! There is little science and much observation. I don't have all the answers and don't pretend to. I hope my ideas stimulate thinking and dialogue that makes us all more effective and more embodying in our work as helpers.

CHAPTER 8

SURVIVAL

SAFETY IN ALL ITS FORMS

One way out of, or better, through the power complex is to
allow spiritual power to move through you, not stay glued
to your ego, where your own needs get in the way.
Thomas Moore[1]

I challenge us all to be able to meet clients in any of their centers,
from any of ours, for the good of their process and their resolution.
Noah Karrasch

This chapter introduces my model of energetic flow in and through head, heart, gut and groin, and considers the physical and emotional health of each center. I believe most of us operate from one or perhaps two of these four major centers, and conversely often shut down in one or more areas, either psychologically or physically, or both. I think we often shut down emotionally first, leading to physical problems later. I also realize a physical trauma can lead to an emotional or psychological pain. (Is this pain psychosomatic, or somatopsychic?) I think and feel this has important implications for the way we both give and receive healing.

Remember I stated in the prologue: I'm not a scientist. I do, however, observe that which is around me, and these next chapters are based on my observations. I find these relationships I discuss in the following chapters are often valid, and I invite us all to look at our own current model to see if these ideas give us new thoughts. This chapter begins the discussion; it doesn't define it!

Stop for a moment to consider two or three people you know with whom being in relationship is difficult. Perhaps you feel in a "one-up" situation, stuck in non-winnable competition with a family member, friend, coworker or boss. Perhaps you're irritated by the "flirty" or "loose" nature some other person in your life seems to send your way, consciously or not. Perhaps you have a needy person in your life who demands constant reassurance. Perhaps your "other" has a different, but equally irritating habit or behavior that makes you want to get away from him or her, even though you know you "should be a better person than that."

Let's ask this model to give us clues as to where this other person's stuck or overactive energy resides. The "one-up" person may live in the head, while the flirt probably lives in or from the groin. The needy person may be blocked in gut or heart. Can we observe this partner's unbalanced spots in relation to our *own* weak, over- or underactive spots? Can we think and feel through how to internally validate and accept self and other without getting activated by their behaviors? Can we learn how to internally validate this self-toward-other as well as this other-through-self? Can we be fulfilled enough to *want* to see others fulfilled in the same measure as we'd like to be in our own core? Can we transfer this talent, this ability to perceive where our patrons' "stuckness" resides, so we can more effectively help them resolve this stuck energy?

The quote that opens this chapter contains much food for thought: Moore introduces an interesting idea by including ego, and, specifically, the ego as the mechanism by which we block energy movement through the centers. Imagine that each of these four emotional or physical centers is also an ego center: Does someone operate from the head ego, the heart ego, the gut ego or the groin ego? Other words might serve—physical or emotional centers, brains, controlling centers—the descriptor is less important. Where do we live? Where do we hide?

The larger concept for me is the idea that ego/energy lives, or hides, anywhere and everywhere, but too often doesn't move freely through the entire system. All of us could be more honest in discerning which of our centers holds the strongest and most powerful egoic congestion. Can we then try to get that ego/energy center on track so that we again operate from all the centers, brains or controls? Can we learn how to stay open to others while validating them—and while staying out of our own fears (usually some form of lack, not enough love)? Can we allow ourselves to *feel* self-validation, so as to offer validation to others without becoming their lifeline and feeling sucked into their well?

We live or hide in any of these ego centers because of old held attitudes or responses to one or more of life's activating events, our trauma or unprocessed information. *Unless bodymindcore awareness can travel freely through this entire geographic four-point system in a balanced fashion, health is compromised.* Weakness, fear, disease: All are congestion. All suggest something is blocked. If we begin to examine both where the block is primary and why we're allowing it to remain, we're moving stuck energy. Recognizing unacknowledged fear and weakness begins the process of reversing and resolving disease or even decay. This flowing or stuck energy concept supports the theory of the "create your disease" believers: We do create our personal life experience, if in no other way than by choosing to hold onto the attitude that any event is a trauma instead of simply an activating event. "...for there is nothing either good or bad, but thinking makes it so."[2]

Earlier in the book I presented the Franks' idea that both demoralization and lack of validation contribute to illness (page 36). Let's begin to consider that each of these four centers needs to feel valid; more specifically, that any or each needs to remove that which makes it feel invalid. Call it trauma, disease or unprocessed information: There's something in one or more centers in all of us that could still be freed, opened, and understood if we're to get better.

Perhaps each too-open or too-closed center is actually searching for its power. Does energy moving through a groin produce pleasure power, or control power? Ask the same question of the gut, the heart, and the head. Answers will give strong cues as to where one might focus healing energy in oneself or in another.

Can we begin to examine which of our personal centers is activated and which is feeling invalidated, both in our helper role and in our personal lives? If we begin to notice recurring energetic blocks and/or leaks in our patron/other, can we use this information to advantage in helping them change their blocks, by examining the relevance of their blocks to our own? If we constantly attract patrons with similar patterns to our own, can we use the information to examine our processes and make changes? I challenge us as practitioners to experiment with finding and feeling these control centers in ourselves, keeping them in better balance one to another, then recognizing them in others. This will help us become more informed and effective helpers. We can examine others with this model, observe which of their centers seems out of balance and how their imbalances relate to our own, and with this knowledge hope to address their issues more honestly, as we more honestly face our own energetic slowdowns.

Remember Sunny Cooper's work referred to in Chapter 4 (see page 63), suggesting how, without awareness, the archetype of any practitioner attracts clients of an archetype that feeds the practitioner's egoic archetype? A head-centered practitioner could be considered a sage; they'll primarily attract seekers, if they're not aware of what they're doing. A heart-centered practitioner, a nurturer, will attract children. A gut-centered practitioner, a rescuer, will attract victims; and a groin-centered practitioner, a magician, will attract destroyers. *Unless*, that is, all these practitioners recognize from which center they primarily operate, and actively work to stay open to all patrons.

Getting self and patrons aware of all four of these centers and learning to operate clearly from any and all of them is an intriguing addition to the future of the creation of health in all of us. As a practitioner partner, I believe it's my responsibility to operate as fully as possible from head, heart, gut and groin, if I am to ethically challenge opening in any of the four centers the patron needs to examine. In our coming work with each center we'll discuss how living in and operating exclusively from, or hiding in, any one center makes us a less effective therapist for the entire group of people who come across our path. This realization of where we live and don't live in our own bodymindcores may show us why we haven't been able to attract a more general patron population, instead of the same client personality type too consistently.

The old truism that "what we focus on expands" applies here; if we're not aware of our limitations and their habits, we'll continue to perpetrate and perpetuate a model that looks for, and finds, a certain kind of neediness in our patrons. We can't establish balance for others if we're busy fortifying our own blockages, and we'll limit our own practice. That overriding patron need will be the need we most like to fulfill, based on our own centers and their energetic blockage or overactivity. So in the next four chapters we'll examine head, heart, gut and groin and the implications of living or not living in each of these important areas. We'll see if we as therapists or practitioners or healing partners can better learn to walk the talk. Again, I hope that we as practitioners can find our energy moving freely through our own centers, so we can better assist others in this energy movement.

In these next chapters I'll share my thoughts about each of the four centers and how they relate to the other centers of the body. I've thought at length about which words I want to use to describe too-open and too-closed centers. My list was long, and I haven't found an appropriate pairing to describe exactly what I'm seeing or seeking. "Active/passive" approaches what I want to say, as does "parent/child"—especially as the parent/child relationship suggests the parent ultimately wants to share an equal relationship with that child. Various pairings convey the concept, but none with quite the tone I wish to share. So I'll stay with the terms open and closed to describe these centers.

Let's use more words to help describe those who are either overactive (or open) in a center, or underactive (or closed). We could see one who is overactive in the *groin* as promiscuous, while one who is closed might be ungrounded and potentially frigid. A person overactive in the *gut* may be over-discerning and perhaps too intuitive; a closed gut is judgmental. A *heart*-centered person is probably nurturing and even over-nurturing, while the closed-heart person seems and feels uncaring. The overactive *head* seems too analytical, while their underactive partner whose head remains closed can appear unfocused and scattered. While these are generalities, it's helpful to see these eight types of person, based on where the energy is overactive or underactive. And you begin already to see how an open head relating to a closed head makes for a difficult relationship.

A brief recapitulation on chakras may be useful here, since many mainstream medical workers haven't taken the opportunity to learn about this system. If you'd like more of my thoughts about chakras, please refer to my book *Freeing Emotions and Energy Through Myofascial Release*.[3] The chakra model comes from India; the Sanskrit word *chakra* means "wheel" or "spin." There are seven major chakras in the body. The lowest and highest have funnels or whirlwinds of energy moving respectively skywards (above) and earthwards (below). The other five chakras have whirlwinds facing both front and back, horizontally.

The first chakra, physically at the perineum between genitals and anus, is the center of survival and safety. Bearing in mind how much of this book is devoted to safety, readers can surmise I find this chakra to be important. Chakra two, located in the band of sacrum and genitals, is sacral/sexual and the location of issues of shame around sex, power and money. In my head/heart/gut/groin model you'll find I've joined these two centers together as "groin."

The third chakra, the solar plexus, located in the stomach, is that area where we discern in the gut, instead of judging in the head. The fourth, or heart chakra is the area that wants us to live with purpose, with our "heart in it." The fifth, the throat, deals with the ability to express creatively (or not, if closed). The sixth, often called the "third eye," is situated between and above the eyes, at the center of the forehead. This is the place where we think and rationalize—all being well, without too much over-thinking, worry and judgment.

The final, seventh chakra is often called the crown and resides slightly above the person's head. I prefer to see this chakra as the "higher self"; some sort of guide that can operate for us from a higher perspective, if we'll only use it. While I think we judge in our heads and discern in our guts, I also believe we make our best decisions by consulting our heads, hearts, guts and groins before ultimately deciding in our higher self.

In this book I'll focus on the first, root or survival chakra only as it relates to the second or sexual/sacral chakra... It's my belief that if one is still on the planet, the lower chakra is sufficiently open. If it wasn't open, one would be dead, or at least, dying rather quickly. Hay and Schulz in *All is Well* suggest, "The health of the first emotional center depends on your feeling safe in the world... If you fundamentally don't believe that you are capable or worthy of receiving support, foundation, and security, medicine alone won't be able to cure what ails you. You must address the underlying beliefs that led you down the road of health problems in the first place."[4] We're back to safety issues, and they clearly are the "root" problem… Until one feels a degree of safety, hoarded energy becomes stuck in the first and second chakra areas. While the first chakra *may* be closed, I find the primary blockage is just above, in the sacral/sexual area. So I place this survival fear in the second, tail-wagging joy and reproduction/creation chakra, instead of in the traditional spot.

Traditional chakra maps show the first and seventh chakras (we'll discuss the seventh chakra in Chapter 13) represented by single funnels or whirlwinds of energy, the first chakra pointing downward and the seventh pointing skyward (instead of double funnels on a horizontal axis, as the other five chakras are). This is yet another reason why I prefer the head/heart/gut/groin model. I see the upper and lower chakras as different, being our connection to the heavens and the earth, whereas the other five centers represent our connections to the environment and our interactions in it—our future and our past. The throat chakra is absent from my four-center formula because I believe the throat remains open when the head and heart are happily and cooperatively keeping their distance from, yet still communicating with one another.

I encourage each of us to become an integrated and integrative health partner—someone who can operate equitably not only from these four centers, but also from the centers above, below, and in the middle of all four (respectively the crown chakra, the higher self or oversoul; the lowest center, the root or survival chakra; and the throat center, which enables creative expression). I challenge us all to be able to meet clients in any of their centers, from any of ours, honestly and cleanly, for the good of their process and their resolution. I encourage us all to recognize which of their centers—and ours first!—are open, too open, closed or too closed, and to learn to move freely and appropriately from center to center in our own bodies as we endeavor to help patrons find balance in their own centers and communicate with them in any and every ego spot.

We can endeavor to coax patrons to fuller awareness of *positive group reality*, which might also be defined as resilience in community or humanity. I'd further suggest this positive group reality is that ability to interface horizontally with others, instead of only with the earth or heavens or self; with any and all aspects of our environment and its occupants, instead of microscopically with only our own cores.

If most of us are "stuck" open *or* closed in one center or another, we as caregivers must each fearlessly examine where *we* live and why we stay there, before we try to make changes in those who cross our paths. The first rule of healing, from the beginning of time to the present day, is: "Physician, heal thyself." If one isn't healthy, what does one truly offer? The second rule most of us try to follow is the Hippocratic Oath: "First, do no harm." It's easy to think we know what's best for someone else; yet probably most of us in healing work have realized on at least a few occasions that our best efforts may actually have harmed another person, no matter how good our intentions. And both of these directions *negate* "Take charge." Too many of us, before we've tried to heal ourselves, and in our desire to take charge of someone else's process, really do them harm.

Too many of us still live on that "unsafe" planet—causing us to flee, fight or freeze. Our primary goal as a helper might still be to coax that health seeker into a safer worldview and enable them to feel their feelings. Too many of us are doing all we can to hold on for the ride whilst stuck in that fear-based mode in which every activating event is a trauma. Where can I hide? Will I survive? How can I survive? What skills and mechanisms help me survive? Why would or should I want to release that defense which has been working for me, especially if its release might jeopardize my survival or destabilize the world I've created to protect me?

Time, process and patience are important factors in finding our healing and guiding others to it as well. Many of us didn't get our trauma in a few seconds, but over time. Most of us have carried our trauma through time and allowed it to take over more and more of our process. Therefore we need patience as we face the time it may take to complete, to release and then resolve our trauma through that process. Maybe we're all afraid of time instead of determined to make the most of it. Maybe true healing is that moment when one realizes that *time isn't the important concept; presence is.* Certainly many, as they approach death, realize and embody that savoring of and living fully in the present moment. Indeed, it may be the final worthwhile activity. Maybe some are healed as they give up life in the body, because ultimately healing is found only in the present moment. Maybe…

Let's now take the time to examine the styles of practitioners whose egos operate from either an underactive, stuck center or an overactive and overbearing one, in any of the four areas—the groin-, gut-, heart- or head-centered (or, alternatively, deprived) practitioner partner. I'd like to look briefly at how these eight types of practitioners (four overactive open "drivers" and four underactive or closed "passengers") relate to clients who are stuck living—or hiding—in the same or different body centers. It's fascinating and challenging to look at who and where we, as caregivers, are and to consider how we consequently relate to clients of varying types and stripes. I believe safety, and therefore health, are expressed in the four centers, as satisfaction (groin), self-esteem (gut), purpose (heart) and clarity (head). Clearly, if and when we can create safety in all four of these centers of the body of another (and first in ourselves), health and healing are much closer than when we allow ourselves or our patrons to remain closed in one or more of these centers, and overactive in others.

Berceli labels these four centers differently in his work, though I'm not sure he'd agree with my juxtaposition: "Situations that threaten our social self such as rejection [I see heart involvement], shame [groin], fear of failure [head], and negative judgment by others [gut] cause us to react in the same manner as if we were being threatened physically."[5] While he's using slightly different words, in some ways, I believe they create a model similar to my own. And remember Cooper's archetypical model (page 63); again, four major centers are featured—Magician at sacral/sex, Rescuer in the solar plexus, Nurturer at the heart and Sage at the head (my juxtaposition, not Cooper's).

I hope that you, the reader, see the value of the practitioner who has already done their own work so as to remove impediments in each of these body segments. Such a practitioner is able to move freely from groin to gut to heart to head, headward and tailward, quickly and easily, as the situation and the client's physical cues suggest which center and which issues are the ones to examine more effectively. Can we meet our seeker where they are and bring them into more of their bodymindcore? This free movement of energy between centers in practitioners, as well as the ability to recognize the feeling both of movement and of getting stuck in one or more areas, seems necessary to me if we're to become better helpers of those who want to change.

While patrons might resonate with this energetic model were it presented to them, more likely they simply want to feel better. Moving energy freely, staying aware of problem centers, helping them to modify behaviors through recognizing our own patterns, and developing the ability to coax others out of, into, and through overactive or stuck bodymindcore centers are *our* goals. Whether a center is underactive or overactive, it's still out of balance, and though it's seeking balance, it's still inappropriate behavior on the part of ourselves as helpers to try to change a patron without being honest about our own blocks.

Peter Levine describes his work as "Somatic Experiencing," and I think it's appropriate to describe in a bit more detail how (it seems to me) he speaks about similar concepts in a slightly different language. Levine encourages us to coax clients back into their body sensations, rather than just looking at feelings. He asks his clients to find the physical blocks and put awareness into them, so the fear, the paralysis of a blocked energy center, what Upledger in craniosacral therapy might call an energy cyst (simply his term for a similar energy blockage), can be released. Levine's work "...helps to create physiological, sensate and affective states that transform those of fear and helplessness. It does this by accessing various instinctual reactions through one's awareness of physical body sensations."[6]

I believe Levine is asking for nearly the same resolution as I want to coax from clients. Put most simply, he encourages his clients to stay in their bodies while they face their fears. For me this model of keeping clients present echoes my belief that too many of us "freeze" or play dead due to our own fears or our overwhelmed bodymindcore state. *Can we encourage and allow our patrons to explore those deep old hurts and restore energy to those parts that have been holding their breath, or haven't bothered to take a breath lately?* This is my overwhelming question and focus as a practitioner partner.

I come at these issues, and most issues, through my training and background as a bodyworker. From that perspective I'm probably most entitled to share these *physical* thoughts and comments. It's probably the reason why Levine's claim that we come best to our healing partners' traumas through the body instead of the mind resonates with me. No matter why a particular center of the body is traumatized, underactive, shut down (or whichever term you prefer), can we choose to remember how to open, activate or at least *be aware of our own blocks* so we can better serve our patrons?

For each of the following four chapters I've created two tables that deal with the particular center of the body featured in that chapter. (As they will be meaningless to some and useful to others, they are presented as Appendix B.) The tables helped me refine my ideas. If a practitioner has eight options of operation (from open or closed head, heart, gut or groin) and we consider that each patron can operate from the same eight positions, this creates 64 combinations of partnership, with attendant complications (or attendant ease). This doesn't even take into consideration that someone closed in the heart is probably living more fully elsewhere, in head, gut or groin...so the permutations are actually more or less endless, leading me almost to believe it's impossible to create generalizations about relationships between patron and practitioner. You may find this information helpful, and you may not. See it as a work in progress, designed to stimulate thought in me and in you.

There will be some generalities—for example, a blocked groin, gut or heart often causes a person to live in the head. A closed head center may cause a person to live lower down, usually in the heart, but possibly also in groin aspects. Many of us are shut down in groin and gut. So this isn't a foolproof model by any stretch. Yet it seems worthwhile to offer guidelines that provide general descriptions of various partnership combinations. I offer these ideas solely for the purpose of helping the practitioner partner look more closely at their *own* patterns, to see if they're truly contributing to their partner's well-being, or if they're actually resonating with that other's congestion. Becoming aware of one's personal open and closed centers and recognizing the same in the patron, gives a practitioner yet another tool to understand why sometimes their sessions succeed and other times they fail.

The tables in Appendix B are meant, first, to be seen as an exploration, not a perfect roadmap. I'm reminded that Ida Rolf reportedly used to quote Dr. Alfred Korzybski: "The map isn't the territory (and the word is not the thing)."[7] It's my intention to create a system that enables a practitioner to examine honestly what's open and what's closed in their own system, compare it with the system of their patron partner, and determine how to proceed most effectively with that patron's process. On occasion I actually feel the recognition of these open and closed centers as they relate to both partners is a warning signal that suggests, "*Proceed with extreme caution.*" An open groin is often one such center.

So the tables and the following four chapters challenge any practitioner to first determine honestly which centers are open or closed in themselves, then to determine the patron's state and see how compatible (or alternatively how dangerous) their partnership with that patron might be. What are the warning signals? What configurations should be avoided, or at least respected and handled carefully?

And one last thought before we move into the main model of interactions: Many of us become either too grounded, but stuck, in lower centers, or too cerebral or nurturing, but stuck, in the upper centers. I see the diaphragm muscle as the stricture of an hourglass, which seems to separate our two beings—the grounded, safety-seeking, lower, earthly body from the head-to-heart, purpose- and thought-driven, upper, heavenly body. How do we as practitioners bridge this gap, operate both in the higher realms and the earthly ones, so as to become better in our work with others, professionally and personally?

In the coming chapters I'll theorize about my observations of bodies in general and the repercussions and symptoms one finds in each specific energy center or chakra—either underactive or overactive. As we move forward into my model of the four energy centers and how they affect us both as humans and as healing partners, I invite you to put aside the judgments that may come up around your own wounds and how they relate to the patrons you attract. Allow yourself to experience these ideas without shame, judgment or anger. Allow yourself to consider whether there may just be something for you in the following pages.

CHAPTER 9

SATISFACTION SAFETY

Therapists can investigate their own longings, desires, and fears around the physical body, physical sex, spiritual sex, touch and vital energy.
Kylea Taylor[1]

According to the Tao, all of the organs and glands in your body give their best energy, what is called orgasmic energy.
Chia and Abrams[2]

It seems to me we're all afraid to honestly examine our sexual energy and allow it to flow through our body.
Noah Karrasch

We begin our view of open and closed centers with the area too many of us try to keep under wraps—the groin. Too often we're afraid to acknowledge or discuss our sexual feelings, fearing they're worthless, injured or in some way not good enough. It's easier to pretend we have no sexual feelings, especially toward our patrons. Perhaps a less fearful examination of our own centers could assist us in learning to coax troubled seekers through their damaged sexual centers.

Hay and Schulz: "…the key to mastering health in this emotional center is learning how to manage your finances without sacrificing your love life and vice versa… For second emotional center problems, we find four types of people: those who would rather focus on love than money, those who focus on money rather than love, those who have an unbridled drive to move forward in money and love, and those who can't responsibly handle either love or money."[3]

I'd suggest that part of what we're hearing from the disparate sources above is that most people with second chakra blocks *or* overactivity (I feel few are balanced and most of us experience one or the other) have either sexual satisfaction issues, or satisfaction issues with their life. Those who would rather focus on love seem to be anchored in the heart and not the groin, while those who focus on money seem anchored in the head and blocked in the groin. Those with the drive to move forward in love and money seem to live from the gut, and those who can't responsibly handle either may live in an overactive groin. Money may or may not be as large an issue in second center activities as feeling *unsatisfied in life*. One could argue that for too many people, money *is* satisfaction. In all of these scenarios, the open or closed groin center signifies issues with satisfaction in life.

Whether sexual or money issues, groin energy revolves around this satisfaction or its lack—the need to seek more, or to repress. Is money satisfaction some people's substitute for sexual satisfaction? I believe it is…We're all dealing with safety and shame issues, and nearly all of us have at least a degree of congestion in this second chakra area. Whether because of early sexual or emotional abuse, physical injuries, inappropriate use of body and mind, or early training that satisfaction is for others but not for us, many become mired in their sexual center. Reich's orgasmic energy is tied in knots: Whether we can't move sexual energy or whether it moves *too* freely through us, we may become dissatisfied. We may not be able to move sexual energy through us (no inbreath, expired), or we may not have enough residual energy due to that too-frequent movement through us (no outbreath, inspired).

The word "shame" can also be used to describe groin feelings and the reason for suppressing them. In my opinion, many of us are still ashamed that we have sexual organs and feelings that course through them. Whether because of abuse issues, self-esteem issues or simply never learning how to live comfortably in our sexual apparatus, we hide from ourselves and our feelings, ashamed. Most of us don't even know what exactly we're ashamed of possibly having done. Can we touch our hiding and shamed patrons without judgment of them or their process, while remaining in a place where we as caregiver constantly remember they're a worthy soul who's paying for our trustworthiness? If we can do that, we need to do so; if we can't do it, we need to move to another profession. A groin's energy needs to be touched, but with a reverence and an intention to cleanly help another move through their blocks, without introducing one's own work or need for power into this other's process.

Generally, most practitioners who try to provide assistance to patrons aren't going to be the magician archetype of Cooper's earlier model, operating from their own overpowering shame and survival center. Therefore they'll probably be able to stay in the field for an entire career. Eventually some ethical dilemma may confront those who haven't worked through or aren't willing to look at personal groin issues as they believe in and practice their magic. This inability to face self may trigger overstepping of boundaries and engaging in inappropriate behavior. We'd prefer to ignore this dilemma because, most probably, a helper with a closed groin isn't usually a problem to their patrons, and one with an open groin is engaging their movement of sexual energy outside their therapy practice (has already been "outed").

We just don't see that many "therapists" or "helpers" anchored and acting out primarily from groin issues. It does happen enough (not necessarily sexually, but maybe in power playing) that we need to examine honestly and acknowledge what's taking place here, and ponder what we can do to change this pattern. I remember a totally unqualified acquaintance in our town who used to "counsel" needy women, with no counseling credential whatsoever and with the rumored intention of finding women to use for his sexual gratification. He was probably the poster child for what can go wrong when a "helper" hasn't been looking at their own issues.

Too many of us are afraid to feel our "inappropriate" sexual and power feelings in whatever may seem to be our accepted group's moral code. We're afraid of "What would they say?" and some of us even provide our own "they." We self-censor and don't allow ourselves to become who we truly want to be, sexually—as "I" and "me" disagree about what's proper. More and more I perceive the battle between "I" who often lives in head or heart, and the elusive "me" who's being hidden *somewhere*—elsewhere, or possibly even in the same place— what Tolle calls "the little me."[4] And you and I have a better chance of working in partnership if my I and my me (possibly my ego and my id?) are able to integrate and communicate with each other.

So most of us are afraid to examine sexual energy honestly and let it flow through our body. We've become obsessed with the idea of perfection: perfect body, perfect partnership, perfect sex and perfect orgasm. I think we'd be better served by learning to enjoy our present body, orgasm, sex and partnership (if there is a partnership with another) instead of waiting for perfect conditions to appear for perfect sex to happen. The *I* and the *me* can better integrate if they agree that the present condition and feeling are not only good enough, but satisfactory, and free of shame.

Chia and Abrams in *The Multi-Orgasmic Man* suggest that sexual energy happens to be stuck in the sex organs, but needs to be moving freely throughout the body: "Sexual energy, or *ching-chi* (pronounced JING-CHEE) in Chinese, is one of the most obvious and powerful types of bioelectric energy… Sexual Kung Fu practices are based on cultivating this sexual energy and using it to increase your overall energy and health. You must learn to draw your sexual energy out of your genitals and to circulate it through the rest of your body to truly master the Taoist techniques for experiencing multiple and whole-body orgasms and for improving your health."[5] These authors affirm again that sexual energy isn't a problem; it's stuck sexual energy that's the problem. When you as the practitioner partner have problems with the movement of your own sexual energy, then, especially if you're overusing the groin, you are an accident waiting to happen with a needy seeker.

Therefore, it seems to me that before we can help to move healthy sexual energy through *any* other body, we need to learn to allow sexual feelings to permeate *our* sexual organs, our root chakra, our survival issues, and then achieve a feeling of satisfaction with those feelings, issues and areas so they can travel upward through the rest of the body and allow energy there as well. We must learn to feel and allow uncensored yet responsible sexual feelings to arise through our lower centers in order to experience that orgasmic energy in higher realms of the body. If this is hard to achieve or currently unavailable with a committed partner, work with the self is entirely appropriate. How can you love someone else, or how can someone love you, if you don't love yourself? How can you love yourself if you won't take the time to feel yourself, your feelings, and your sexual energy, and allow that orgasmic energy to permeate you?

Most massage schools spend a great deal of time, and rightly so, instilling the ethical idea that massage as a career is not a place for someone with sexual issues. Students are taught early that several places on the body are "no-no's," and if many clients want to be touched "down there," or if a student believes they're ready to touch others in such a spot, chances are they need a different profession.

Yet, it's amazing to me how much good work I and others have been able to do in the first and second chakra areas—the shameful sexual–sacral–survival safety repository. If patron and practitioner are able to remain detached from the emotional bond that's undoubtedly forged when two people become this intimate—if both can remain clinical, neutral and empathic—amazing changes for the better can happen in patrons. If the practitioner respects the power granted to them, the patron can receive healing—physical, mental and emotional, as well as chemical and energetic changes, in my practical experience.

Too many of us seem too afraid to look honestly at, and without judgment touch, the most private safety issues of our *other*, issues the patron can be hiding and guarding, or recklessly trying to face, set free, or learn to control. When we get our hands or intention below a belly, we're playing with fire—literally. In the Oriental medicine model we're challenging or coaxing the seeker to consider allowing the groin's burner to heat the belly's *dantian* or energy center in a way that can send energy on up to heat the heart's energy and fuel the brain, and on to the higher self—a worthy goal. We're asking a large percentage of our patrons, whether their complaint is in the low body or not, to allow the movement of life energy to flow up and out of the earth's artesian well and actually irrigate the parched and tight areas above: in the heart, in the neck and shoulders, in the arms and hands. This is Reich's orgasmic energy, the *chi* of the total bodymindcore and the magic of a true magician.

Let's experiment. Lie on the floor or a bed, on your back. Extend first one heel and straight leg as far away from the hip as possible, while jamming the other heel *with a straight leg* as close as you can toward the tailbone. Then extend the tightened leg/heel, pressing the formerly lengthened heel and straight leg as close as you can to your tailbone. Next, focus on keeping the low back down into the floor as you extend the heel, while breathing and putting awareness into your pelvic floor and low belly. Can you allow yourself to find the pelvic area and feel energy stirring there? Too many of us are afraid of what we might find, and so don't allow any flow in the pelvis. (This and several other awareness ideas are featured together in Appendix A.)

I've been rereading several of Scott Peck's books and finally found a particular quote I remembered from nearly 30 years ago, in which I believe he tried to initiate this very conversation. In *The Road Less Travelled*[6] he suggested, to quite a bit of negative feedback, that he might have sex with a client if he believed it was appropriate and enhanced the client's healing process. He affirmed he'd never allowed this particular situation to come to reality, but he wasn't certain that it might not at some point happen.

This idea stayed with me, partly because of fears of my own sexual insecurities and how they might spill out to others, and partly because of the total taboo he was admitting might have exemptions. As I revisit his concept in this day, I marvel that someone could feel enough mastery of their own sexual center and its need for power that they could believe they'd be able to engage in sex with this other and not muddy the waters of that other's process and health, as well as complicate their own. I'm still pondering this position.

To me, those who believe they can control their sexual energy appropriately while severely challenging the sexual energy of another are too often lying to themselves. If they're honest, they'll admit they're serving their own needs more than their clients' healing. This is true not only in the sexual realm! Nearly any touch to anyone can be about our need to improve or enhance ourselves at the expense of our clients or patrons, if we're not aware and very careful. I can't imagine feeling so totally complete in my own sexual energies that I would truly believe I'd be helpful to a seeker by joining sexually as part of a healing process.

In *The Ethics of Caring*[7] Taylor says, "Most ethical issues in ordinary therapy with clients concern money, sex, and power. Although most professional codes of ethics do not use the headings money, sex, and power to list their guidelines, most of the ethical principles listed concern these areas." I believe all three live in, get stuck in, or can't get through, the groin. Money and its accumulation are about power; too much of sexual relationship involves power. Generally when someone uses sex or money irresponsibly, they want power. And when any "therapist" decides they must control the process of a client, they've become "the-rapist."

In the past I've taught ethics courses to massage therapists— not because I believed I had any ethical magic pills to dispense, but because the course was required and someone was needed to teach it. As a teacher of ethics, my first question to self was: "What do I teach?" I decided to review the counseling code of ethics and find similarities and differences and move forward from what was already being done.

In addition to common-sense bits in the counseling codes, such as not creating or accepting dual relationships, maintaining confidentiality, being self-policing as a community, and notifying authorities if there is clear and present danger to a client or others, the elephant in the livingroom always seemed to be the inappropriate creation of sexual relationships. Most people didn't seem to have problems accepting confidentiality, self-policing or other codes. In most classes I'd have one female student who confided that many male clients approached her sexually. It was intriguing to see other students look at this particular student with knowing eyes: "Somehow, you're doing this to yourself."

It's true, I believe. If you as a therapist continue to have issues with patrons who are attracted to you and who try to act on that attraction, it's not all about the client! There's still some old habit in your closet that puts a sign on your forehead saying "available" or "touch/don't touch." The first, most important step in this situation is to admit this is so; otherwise, one keeps attracting patrons who keep pushing the same buttons the healing partner has been working so hard to disarm in self by touching others' vulnerabilities. If you are such a one, stop!

In some classes I'd also have one or two students who insisted the group ethics code we wrote at the end of the course must include specific statements about not participating in sexual activities. It seemed that in these instances I often detected students who'd been wounded or abused in their sexual energy center at some earlier time in their life, possibly in a therapeutic setting, and so felt this specific instruction must be spelled out for all. They strongly felt that, otherwise, silence on the subject implied permission to therapists to touch inappropriately.

Sometimes I believe we all "wear our heart on our sleeve." It seems that both the groups above are coming either from the overactive groin that silently signals to the patron availability for sexual contact, or from a closed, "don't touch" groin that needs delineation no matter how many behaviors are codified as inappropriate. Practitioners neither too open nor too closed in their groin usually don't care what's said in such a written code. If some patron does approach them inappropriately, they deal with the transgression swiftly and decisively, without recourse to a written code.

So, clearly, a practitioner who is still stuck in either too-open or too-closed groin issues may attract patrons who are also working to resolve groin issues. This is potentially a recipe for disaster. I don't know of many situations of therapists who have allowed such a relationship to develop who haven't regretted their indiscretion. Have they learned from it? Let's hope so. Have they grown through it? That remains to be seen. Has it been therapeutic for the patron? Doubtful. Is it truly possible to have therapeutic sex with that "other," the patron, without damaging that patron's process, and possibly one's own as well? I can only answer for myself—I'm not that advanced yet.

I believe a practitioner partner stuck in an overactive groin might actually be a suitable match for a patron who lives in their head; perhaps they could help to ground this individual and bring them down to earth a bit more. This is probably the only fairly safe combination of practitioner and patron when the practitioner lives in an overactive groin, however. Any patron may face disaster if dealing with a practitioner living in an open groin. Groin energy may awaken the patron into their own groin as well. A patron who's already floundering in their stuck sexual energy, either too open or too closed, absolutely doesn't benefit from a "therapist" who is working through their own stuck sexual needs by dealing with the sexual energy of others. A destroyer doesn't truly need help from a magician so much as from a rescuer or a nurturer or a sage—someone who will get them back in touch with their upper body. And while many practitioners may allow themselves to believe they're actually helping such a patron, their head—if they'd allow themselves to check as high up the line as the head—would know this for the falsehood it is.

So, should people who are overactive in the groin work on others? As in the massage schools I've mentioned above, I hope their school and/or accrediting agencies have noticed their behaviors and kept them from practicing until they've faced their own issues and made more appropriate choices. If not, this is where I believe each profession does need to maintain the self-policing code counselors pledge to uphold. It's a disaster to us all when a practitioner is wired only to move energy through their groin. Such a practitioner is a hazard to him- or herself, to the patron, to the profession, and to their local community.

I like what Taylor has to say regarding this use or misuse of sexual energy between caregiver and client: "If the caregiver acts on his own attraction or the client's in an external way, it can divert the client's focus from the internal movement of the client's energy. The process, which is really an internal psychospiritual process, is subverted when the caregiver encourages sexual contact to fulfill his personal needs... Clients who trust a healer or a spiritual teacher feel injured when that person puts his own needs ahead of his client's best interests."[8] I agree with Taylor: The worst gift we can present to a patron is our own, unresolved sexual stuff. Some few of us are still trying to move our own stuck energy through our patrons' processes. Practitioners who want to work on their own sexual energy issues need to do it with a trained professional, not with needy patrons.

But what about that *underactive* groin center in a practitioner? First, in my thinking, these partners tend to be more judgmental;

as they can't reach their own groins, they're blocked in the groin and often living in their head. Their energy often won't flow freely through the body into the groin, and they're more fear-based. They can function in the world, and many do a fair job of fooling the rest of us. They live vicariously through their patrons instead of feeling their own sexual energy or the movement of energy through their own bodies. The only movement of energy they truly feel may be their patron's energy. This practitioner may be doing good work, and may get good results. However, it seems they're living a sham if they won't find their own survival and shame centers and work to move energy through them, but choose to work on the energy centers of others instead.

So this closed groin practitioner could often be called an "open head center" practitioner, from where they will do adequate work. Dealing with a heart-centered patron when one comes from the head, for example, may be difficult but not dangerous. Likewise head-to-head or head-to-gut connections may not be the most effective, but don't have as many caution flags waving; there's the potential for a safe meeting of the two centers in this pairing.

Occasionally, it's possible these closed groin practitioners will come across someone who stirs in their sexual energy a feeling of desire. Disaster! Those who spend time making sure they repress their sexual energies may eventually have problems nearly as big as those who live in an overactive groin. That which we resist, persists.

The bottom line: As practitioners, we must look honestly at our own sexual issues and shortcomings and be realistic about them before delving into the sexual energies of others. If a practitioner expends much energy thinking about sex, participating in sex, or believing most of their patrons need attention in sexual centers, chances are that practitioner has work to do in their own sexual center before touching others. If someone has no sexual energy through their own bodymindcore, chances are they won't be a dangerous practitioner; just not as effective as they might be had they done their own work. We'll return to this sexual issue a bit later in Chapter 12, as we discuss what it means to be stuck living from the head.

CHAPTER 10

SELF-ESTEEM SAFETY

Judge not, that ye be not judged.
Bible (King James Version)[1]

*A practitioner partner who hasn't yet moved into his / her gut
energy (and there are multitudes!) is often more interested in
fixing those "out there" as opposed to looking "in there."*
Noah Karrasch

"Judgment" is an intriguing word. While Jesus tells us we're better without judgment, Peck suggests: "Jesus did not mean we should never judge our neighbor… What he meant was that we should judge others only with great care, and that such carefulness begins with self-judgment."[2] To me, all interpretations suggest that any judgment other than self-judgment is inappropriate, and more helpful than judgment in any situation is true discernment. I believe judgment lives in the head and true discernment resides in the gut.

Recall Porges' contention that 90 percent of vagus fibers travel back to the brain, relaying the body's messages to the head. This suggests nine-tenths of our bodymindcore information comes from the body; yet too many of us want that 90 percent of the body's received and processed messages to be judged by the brain. We forget to honor the older gut brain that can and should override the information overwhelm we often get simply by trying to remain effective on this planet, in our head. (Remember my "Too Much Information Syndrome" in Chapter 1 (page 26)?) I suggest a practitioner with an open gut is well on the way to being an effective partner, especially if they can access heart and head in addition to operating in and from an open gut. This allows them to honor both afferent and efferent nerve channels and use both sets of information in decision-making—the intuitive gut and rational head brains.

This gut brain is born out in Gladwell's review of research showing that conclusions based on too much information cause people to make poorer decisions than instinctual, snap judgments produce.[3] Berceli verifies this thesis: "During trauma, the body places a priority on the abdominal-pelvic brain over the cranial brain."[4] In some primal way, our guts and their perspective orientation are meant to overrule our heads and their obsession with detail! A practitioner who disavows the gut is probably overriding their discernment in favor of the head's judgment.

If the gut center represents this older, discerning knowing, someone who's underactive and unaware in the gut may be prone to making decisions by way of gathering *too much* information. Such a person can be judgmental in their own style, probably based on information filtered through low self-esteem. How can this ungrounded practitioner, who is probably most comfortable living/hiding in their head, be helpful to a head-centered patron who needs reflective discernment instead of someone else's judgment? How can they truly meet in the heart? How can a gut-blocked practitioner support a heart-centered patron without assuming dominance, when their head is falsely directing their gut to tell them what's right for that seeker? One's gut may feel right for self (if one can hear it), but usually has no business making a discernment as to what's definitively right for another, particularly if one is still actually blocked in one's own gut center and therefore not truly reflecting accurately.

A practitioner who operates more fully from an open gut might resonate greatly with a patron either anchored and active in the groin (as many are), or buried and underactive in the gut (as many more are, and don't even realize). So a gut practitioner dealing with a groin or gut patron block still has a delicate balance to maintain. It's so easy to sympathize and empathize at the gut-level! Any time we allow ourselves to truly tune into the patron's issues, fears and hopes that are anchored in gut or groin, we tread on dangerous ground. It's easy to move from empathy to sympathy—to jump right into the well with the drowning patron. It's also easy to allow our open gut to resonate with a needy patron's groin—open or closed.

Any open-gut practitioner dealing with an open-gut patron may be able to get some of the best work accomplished; both truly want to discern what's right, and listen to internal guidance. And great work can be accomplished when a practitioner lives primarily in an open gut and a patron lives primarily in an open heart—if they'll both make that small leap, understanding can appear. Even when the patron has a closed heart, an open gut has a better chance of coaxing energy into the discerning area. Gut-anchored and discerning may be the best position for a practitioner.

When an open gut center practitioner deals with a heart- or head-centered patron, again gut-level honesty can be a grounding, down-to-earth type of energy that will help that head or heart person reclaim their own gut and groin energy. This is another fine balance, however. Many a caregiver allows their own gut to get "tied in knots" due to their own self-esteem issues. They may have a hard time staying detached from the issues presented by a patron's gut or groin, as well as by a heart or head. Too many patrons who primarily *hide* in the gut, center of discernment, may allow their head or center of judgment to overrule their gut's discernment, and be unable to descend to their gut-level feelings...for them, safety lives in the head.

A practitioner who has gut-level reactions to a heart or head patron can exhibit the empathy that's the external validation, allowing that head or heart patron to feel safe in their lower body. A patron who lives in the head often has a better command of verbal messaging, and a gut-centered practitioner may not be able to articulate to that head what they know at gut-level. A gut-centered practitioner who realizes they have trouble verbalizing to a head patron what they know in their gut is better prepared to deal with such a patron. A patron who lives more in the heart center will often grasp the gut-level concepts such a practitioner presents to them.

What happens if a practitioner hasn't yet found their own gut energy? Such a practitioner partner (and there are multitudes!) is often more interested in fixing those "out there" as opposed to looking "in there." Since they can't be discerners, they may become judges. Their relation to all groins or guts and any closed heart is more difficult. If they can't or won't understand how censored thoughts and feelings need to be examined and processed in oneself before working this process with others, they're being dishonest. An underactive gut often suggests an overactive head that blocks the gut's wisdom, rationalizing what's best for others without necessarily knowing what's best for self.

Remember the earlier discussion around the question, release vs resolve? Could it be possible that too many of us process in our heads, possibly releasing, but don't visit our gut, where resolution might occur? Can we live in the entire body?

A healing partner stuck at their own gut-level seems to be less threatening to any patron than one who is stuck in the groin issues. This may be partly because, if indeed the gut holds self-esteem issues, that practitioner partner gives their all to their patron in an effort to boost their own self-esteem. Yet it's hard to instill self-esteem in others if we don't yet possess it in our own being.

Chances are good a practitioner closed at the gut lives more in heart or head; if so, they may well not get into trouble with patrons with groin issues. It's not a perfect formula, but most of us who won't let ourselves find our gut discernment are trapped in judgment, from where it's harder to get pulled into a patron's groin. But it could happen that a closed gut gets pulled into a patron's open groin. And a closed-gut practitioner working with a closed-gut patron may not get to real issues, but may instead want to release instead of resolve, as both are quite possibly more open at the head. If a patron has an open gut while the practitioner has a closed one, they'll simply have trouble finding common ground.

Hay and Schulz talk of the need to create health in the gut because this emotional center "...is all about an individual's sense of self and how they fulfill responsibilities to others...People with health issues of the third emotional center generally fall into four categories: those who define themselves by focusing completely on the needs of others, those who bolster their sense of self by looking to career and material possessions, those who give up all concept of self and turn to a higher power for support, and those who avoid looking at themselves through feel-good distractions."[5] As

I look at the four categories here, I see those who focus on the needs of others as operating primarily from the heart center, those who focus on career as coming from the head, those who look for a higher power to run things as living primarily in the crown while ignoring the gut, and those who choose the feel-good route as living from the groin. And it seems to me that many of us have a tighter channel between groin and gut than perhaps anywhere…energy just doesn't want to flow easily between the two centers for too many of us.

In other words, nearly all of us have issues in this gut emotional center! Remember, I see this as true partly because nearly all of us have blockages in the groin directly below; thus our energies can't move up and through groin and gut. This is as true of most "therapists" as it is for the general population, I believe. It's hard to find someone who doesn't have at least a few knots left in their stomach, especially if we see energy rising through the body from the earth and survival, up through the groin before it can even reach the stomach on its way to the crown. No one expects any of us to have resolved all the knots in our own guts before working with others. Yet if we create self-esteem in ourselves by focusing on others, on possessions, on our higher power or on addictions, we're not doing self or patron that much good. We're still not doing our own work so much as pretending to do it through our interventions with others.

Consider: Lie on the floor, press your fingertips into your low belly just above the pubic bone, and gently and slowly drag them, fairly deeply, up the front of your spine, through your stomach, and toward your ribcage and costal arch. Intend to bring lower body energy higher in the body. Stay present and breathe deeply. Feel the rise of energy and the feelings in your groin that emanate from that rise of energy. Allow those feelings to be good feelings, and allow yourself to enjoy those good feelings throughout your body. Go slowly, experiment with allowing both breath and awareness to rise with your fingers. As you gently proceed through the stomach, stop and experience the feelings you usually hold inside your gut or groin. (This awareness exercise is also found in Appendix A.)

Consider what we're trying to accomplish with this bit of self work. Realize too many of us with closed groins have a stricture or hourglass that separates the energy of groin from the rest of the body. Simply touching our own bellies with awareness allows us to begin thinking of moving energy farther up the body, to gut, then to heart and head. Can we physically and emotionally dissolve this too-common block with awareness and intention? Work to begin raising energy headward from your groin, then your gut, and toward your heart.

You've actually experimented with an aspect of what some would call a Mayan stomach massage, sometimes called Arvigo therapy (though Arvigo's work is primarily for women),[6] and which probably goes by other names in other cultures. Stay with this stomach awareness process as long as you can: This is a true deep work. The more any one of us stays with this gut energy, works to feel its sensations and hear its messages and entertains the notion of freedom and release through the area, the more resolution of disorder and disease in any of the centers above or below it is enhanced. We'll get healthy if we'll just flush out some of our gut-level fear! This is one interpretation of the work of Pierre Pallardy, presented in *Gut Instinct: What Your Stomach is Trying to Tell You.*[7] Gut work may be the most necessary *and* most difficult work for most practitioners. Those who prefer to live in their head may not even see the validity of this model at all.

Too many of us are afraid to be honest around our first and second centers, groin and gut. Honesty doesn't require that we share these centers physically; it does require that we acknowledge our own blocks and needs and tailor sessions to respect our shortcomings and personal process, without injecting ourselves into the processes of our patrons. As Taylor says in *The Ethics of Caring*: "Therapists can investigate their own longings, desires, and fears around the physical body, physical sex, spiritual sex, touch and vital energy."[8] Investigate, admit, move through those longings, desires and fears. Effective healing work asks for nothing less.

CHAPTER 11

PURPOSE SAFETY

*The future promises fulfillment. That's why
everybody is running towards it.*
Ekhart Tolle[1]

*What I do in reality, is simply hold a space. I allow the
client to determine the direction he or she needs to go.*
Rod Buckner[2]

*The larger caveat for a heart-centered practitioner is their
desire to absorb too much of the energy, the pain, the
blockages from the patron—to become the "sympath."*
Noah Karrasch

Many, perhaps most, practitioners are anchored in or at least comfortable in their hearts. The more "medical" the model from which they operate, the more they may live in their heads instead. But lots of massage therapists, counselors and alternative practitioners primarily anchor themselves in their heart area. If, instead of "seeing" and "hearing" (head-centered) or "understanding" (gut-centered) what one tells them, they "feel" it, chances are they're heart-centered. Potentially, this center and the gut are the best from which to be governed. If the heart center is about purpose and creating safety of purpose, it's rewarding when one feels as a practitioner that one is doing right and perfect work with others. As Moore says, "On the other hand, when soul is present, when you are capable of being present as a human being and making a connection to a patient, even simple applications of your skills will make your work fulfilling and bring you close in touch with the people who come to you for help."[3] If our primary goal is to create safety in patrons, coming from the heart must be the right way to go, right? Clearly we fulfill the Franks' first qualification of caring for our patrons.

Well, perhaps. The large caveat for a heart-centered practitioner is their desire to absorb *too much* of the energy, the pain, the blockages from the patron—to become a "sympath." So the goal for this practitioner is to rein in the amount of sympathy given; to temper it with empathy, thereby not allowing self to get pulled into the tribulations the patron lives—to remember to stay anchored in the head so as to keep an overview of how much energy is being given by the heart.

Hay and Schulz define the heart-centered model thus: "The secret to mastering health in your fourth emotional center is learning how to express your own needs and emotions while also taking into consideration the needs and emotions of others…you need to examine how you maintain your own emotional health while nurturing the emotional health of a relationship."[4] True words, especially for a caregiver who wants to remain clean, yet helpful and empathic, not sympathetic. I'm reminded of Scott Peck's definition of evil as seeking control of others in order to ignore one's own need for spiritual growth. This may be a key thought in the context of this chapter…are we truly trying to grow and evolve ourselves? Are we abusing the trust of the patron? Are we relating in a rescuer mode, or a coaching/cheerleader mode? Or, as Louise Hay suggests, can we become an "emotional midwife"?[5] Can we coax and elicit without overlaying our over-nurturing agenda for our patrons onto their template?

The model I've been developing over the years, to return to my bodywork roots, incorporates the idea that the dome of the diaphragm muscle serves as the floor of the heart and the ceiling of the gut. It's the membrane that keeps them separate. Many diaphragms are in trouble in our society today—as we hold our breath, afraid to inhale and exhale, the muscle becomes tense and/or weakened as a result. Generally I believe we'll find tension in the area and the muscle. I envision an hourglass whose stricture is the top of that diaphragm dome—the stricture is actually the hiatuses, or openings, for aorta, vena cava and esophagus. It behooves us to help our patrons raise their orgasmic energy past their groin and gut and into and through their hearts. I want to tap the sand of this "stuck" hourglass so as to allow gut and heart to communicate, always. While sand runs downhill, realize we can turn the hourglass over; sand needs to run in both directions through this stricture.

This work of asking gut and heart to reconnect also impacts directly on the vagus nerve, my "nerve of well-being," which descends through the neck from the cranium in the carotid channel, moves through much of the chest and stomach cavity in varied branches, and is anchored in the psoas muscle so must move through this tight psoas/diaphragm channel or stricture. While I believe this release of breath and diaphragm can be done with words and intention, I coax with bodywork tools and allow myself to intuit how other actions may encourage this movement of energy toward and through the heart center. Current research on breathing and its effect on heart rate variability demonstrates how a well-developed, mobile diaphragm contributes to overall well-being (see page 33).

I consider the diaphragm muscle and the pelvic floor as two ends of a balloon; what happens in one end affects and is affected by the other. So when the diaphragm tightens, the pelvic floor follows. When we hold our breath, we hold our pelvic floor; if we've tightened our pelvic floor, we're holding our breath. I'm always interested in helping patrons realize they've tightened one or both ends of their balloon. I've got to check into my own balloon to make sure it's *their* bodymindcore I'm trying to loosen, and not my own. And if we tighten gut and groin, we're probably moving energy towards our head.

We may see not only many heart conditions and diseases in patrons, but also fibromyalgia, post-traumatic stress disorder, lung issues and gastric issues such as reflux (or GERD: Gastroesopheogeal Reflux Disease) to name a few. When energy can't move or rise through this stricture between gut and heart, the body is seriously unhappy, and most of us live with at least a mild degree of this constriction. Remember, if energy can't rise through the sexual area or the solar plexus, it probably can't move freely into and through this heart area. Too many of us are stuck, *somewhere.*

Let's try to allow gut energy to rise even further, toward the heart. Roll up a towel, or place a pillow on the floor, and lie on it with the bolster or pillow at about the tenth rib, or halfway up your spine—the bottom of your most forward curving part of spine. Bring your chin toward your chest while the back of your neck stays long. Focus literally on "opening your heart" by trying to pop open a too-shortened front of spine in the heart hinge area. As you breathe, work to visualize the front of your body around the heart getting more open, freer and energized. Can you move energy to the heart? Think of so many of our daily activities: computing, sitting, driving, detail work. Realize how much time we spend pushing ourselves into a fetal position and closing our own "heart hinge" which stops the energetic flow between gut and heart. (You'll find this awareness exercise in Appendix A as well.)

Alternatively, lie face down on the floor with your legs, pelvis and elbows centrally aligned on the floor. Lift your head up and off the floor in a backward tilt while your elbows hold your upper body weight off the ground. Hands can be on the floor in front of elbows, or in the air closer to the head. With stretching and breathing you should feel a bit of opening in this heart/diaphragm area. A very important spot! Can you feel the emotions stirring from this small bit of work?

While both head and heart reside above this main stricture, a heart-centered practitioner can have a great deal of trouble relating to a head-centered patron, as they simply can't understand why someone would live in their thoughts and ignore their feelings all the time. Simply being aware of being heart-centered helps one, as practitioner, to learn to accept head-centered patrons, and even deal with them more effectively. It can also enhance the heart-centered practitioner's ability to coax head-centered patrons to descend further into themselves. The practitioner, meanwhile, can learn to let their own heart energy rise to the head and meet the patron on the level where they live. Learning to live in all four centers and be able to move freely between them continues to make sense.

Heart to heart would seem to be the easiest configuration for both practitioner and patron, and in some ways it can be. However, the larger issue here goes right back to getting sucked into the patron's world, thoughts, feelings, behaviors. Can the practitioner maintain that boundary, that detachment, that's critical to good therapy and good relationship? A heart-centered practitioner is potentially in the best position of any healing partner who is "stuck" in one of the four centers. If you're going to be stuck at all, the heart is probably the best place for it if you want to be of service to others. A heart-centered practitioner dealing with a heart-centered patron can clearly meet that person in a "heart-to-heart" way that can potentially heal both. The challenge still is not to allow one's self to become overwhelmed by the other's heartaches.

A heart-centered practitioner who allows self to get pulled into a patron's groin issues may well have troubles down the line. Our hearts really do bleed for others who are in pain! How can we maintain that professional distance that enables us to remember we're there for the hour, not to assume the path of that person? How can we not let our heart ache for a patron's groin-centered anxiety, their age-old fears and dissatisfactions? How can we not feel heartache for a sexual abuse survivor who really only wants to feel intimacy with someone—anyone—and has built trust for us alone? Can we discern where, apart from the groin, that patron lives, and meet them there? Or conversely realize the patron lives in the groin, and decide *not* to meet them there?

Potentially, an open-heart practitioner working with a gut-centered patron can be fulfilling, if they can transcend that hourglass stricture, that division between the upper and lower body. With either an open or closed heart in the patron, an open heart in the practitioner goes a long way in encouraging exchange of energy. The only fairly easy combination of practitioner head to patron gut is the closed head center of practitioner as it relates to the open gut of the patron. If the practitioner can't reach their own head, they have a "head" start in getting down to the lower center issues.

What about a practitioner who has a "hardened" heart? In what I think of as the oldfashioned current medical system, this might still be a desirable personality. If the heart center is about safety of purpose, someone who seems to have a hard heart can be absolutely on their correct path with a slightly differently calibrated heart barometer... they're not less caring, just differently caring. But I think that unless we are living in our own heart center (or at least know how to be comfortable there) it will be difficult—as it is for me, and most of the practitioners I see—to genuinely care about people enough to fully honor them as we try to help unwind them. The work of Frank and Frank, quoted earlier, shows how feeling cared about as a patron and a person always figures into the equation of getting patrons to feel better. The more we feel connected to others in a non-threatening way, the better we usually feel.

Potentially even a practitioner with a blocked heart center can work well with either an open or a closed patron gut center, though it's difficult. If a blocked heart lives in the head in both partners, the aware practitioner can challenge both to descend and coax both to move further down; if the patron has an open heart while the practitioner is closed there, ideally this practitioner partner has the skill to transcend their own blocks. These can be some of the most frustrating connections. But it's possible for a practitioner with a blocked heart center to resonate with patrons who are either open or closed in their head center.

As you can see, all these combinations and permutations are merely suggestions; there will be no hard and fast rules, and much of what's generalized here is dependent on the skills of the caregiver in recognizing where they allow their own blocks to get in their way. The challenge I wish to raise for us all is to not only recognize our own blocks, but to explore more fully where the patrons' blocks are, so we can transcend them, match their styles and communicate more fully.

Recall my *Twilight Zone* episode when the son became the sin-eater (see page 94). He ate the food from his father's corpse, ate the sins, and assumed the mantle of sin-eater, much to the agony of his mother. This image stuck in my head: As heart-centered therapists, we're most prone to taking on such sins too much of the time! So, be it heart to head, heart to heart, heart to gut or heart to groin: To me, this center is a duality. The place where some of the best work as a practitioner comes, but also the place with the most potential for mismanagement, misunderstanding and therefore damage to both practitioner and patron, is this heart center. This is the place where we can most become a sympath instead of an empath.

CHAPTER 12

CLARITY SAFETY

*To be fully human we must be able to imagine others' hurt and
to relate it to the hurt we would experience if we were in their
place. Consideration is imagination on a moral track.*

P.N. Forni[1]

*If we can't allow ourselves the wisdom of the entire body,
are we able to truly provide service to others?*

Noah Karrasch

Many therapists or practitioners live in their heads. A psychotherapist
may be in their element here; many go into the work primarily
because of the help they've received in dealing with their processes,
and they want to pass on this good work. If we as a caregiver received
our best work through the head because we were open in our head
center, we'll probably want to practice in this head model. While
this is a worthy goal, head-centered practitioners have often reasoned
through their problems and learned to deal with them (release), yet
sometimes don't embody their own work of keeping a clear energetic
channel from groin to head (resolve). Their head may have things
figured out and they may exhibit clarity, but often their hearts, guts
and groins haven't caught up with the work that's been done in and
by the head. While this "head to head" therapy may be satisfying
for both practitioner and patron, is it actually fostering resolution,
or simply accepting release? Are we actually cleaning the closet, or
just making an inventory of the goods? While such therapy can be a
satisfying experience, is it a healing one?

Various countries and sections of the world display different
cultural patterns. In some ways, Americans in particular and westerners

in general tend to live more in their heads; again, I believe, because we don't want to touch the unsafe ground under us. In Asian cultures there seems to be a unity with nature, a groundedness that allows people to live more fully in their lower body centers. Berceli tells of a Japanese student who pointed out to him that, while many Americans commit suicide by shooting themselves in the head, most Japanese commit hari-kari by running a sword through their belly. They believe they kill the spirit or life force in the belly, while Americans believe they kill the life force through the head.[2]

I'm reminded of another quote from Thomas Moore in *Care of the Soul in Medicine* when I think about a head-centered practitioner: "Health care workers…are very rational. They are proud of their methods, the rigor of their education and research, and their strong hold on what they consider reality, which doesn't give much credence to imagery. So in this regard there can be a significant gap between the professional and the patient. We want to help people go through their illnesses and live happy and creative lives… My concern is that evidence-based medicine may become yet another form of impersonal, science-dominated health care… Where is the soul in evidence-based medicine?"[3] And I recall Alan Watts, in *The Wisdom of Insecurity*: "…we have been taught to neglect, despise, and violate our bodies, and to put all faith in our brains. Indeed, the special disease of civilized man might be described as a block or schism between his brain…and the rest of his body."[4] Exactly! This so well affirms my point that too many of us metaphysically reside in the penthouse suite of a four-story condo and never leave that upper story.

As I ponder both of the quotes above, I think of far too many doctors, psychotherapists and scientists who live totally in their heads, discounting the wisdom of the heart and gut. They have the clarity of safety in their heads, but what about the rest of their bodies? Are they safe in the other centers? If we can't allow ourselves the wisdom of the entire body, are we truly able to provide service to others? Do they really care about others? I recently participated in an online chat where the host said something to this effect: "Don't tell me what you're doing works if you can't tell me *why* it works!" I heard a second statement following that one: "Don't bring me a problem if you don't have a solution." My immediate response was, "Why not?" We're back to riding a bicycle with only one wheel if we discount our intuition, our gut brain, in favor of head knowledge alone.

A head-centered therapist may relate easily and well to another "head" but have severe difficulties relating to a heart, gut or groin client. Someone who lives and feels in their heart may or may not be able to hear someone who operates from their head...*there are truly different languages in each center.* My experience has been that those who live primarily in their heads are less able and less interested in moving into the rest of the body; they want neither to feel nor to express that which can't be mentally processed. If it can't be identified and labeled, they're less interested in it and may be resistant to thinking about it.

Hay and Schulz again: "...the health in this center depends on how well you are able to take in information from all realms—both earthly and mystical—and use this information in your life. It depends on how flexible your mind-set is and how you can learn from perspectives different from your own...[head center] health involves a capacity to be receptive to information and a flexibility to think and reason your way out of situations."[5] "Earthly and mystical" suggests we not only move between head/heart/gut/groin, but also down into survival (earthly) and up into caring (mystical) thriving, as well as opening the throat to express all we see and feel.

Hay and Schulz seem to offer us hope here: If you allow yourself to be flexible and receptive to the other centers of the body, to "perspectives different from your own" within your own body, this head center can actually do great work. The problem remains, how do we bring those who live primarily in their heads into the rest of their bodies? In other words, can we learn to allow our emotional elevator to visit all floors: head, heart, gut and groin?

From a physical and bodywork perspective, much of the trouble I see with heads is the fact that they live too far ahead of the body they're supposed to be serving. Whether it's because of physical causes such as too much computer work or detail work, sitting in recliners, believing that old age should make one stoop forward, or feeling unsafe and so pulling the head into its shell so real or imaginary blows from behind won't hurt so much—shoulders and necks are tight because heads are too far forward. The hourglass between gut and heart is mirrored by the one between heart and head—the throat. If we tap this secondary hourglass, the throat chakra is opened, the head fits on top of the body, the heart is opened and expressed, and energy flows. I'm reminded that Ida Rolf is reputed to have told clients that even if they didn't have time for bodywork, they could self-correct by reminding themselves to keep their head up and their waist back. It does seem to help open both these major strictures between centers.

A head-centered healing partner will demonstrate clarity, and so will probably be very good at talking with the client, at probing them with the appropriate words and metaphors, but may imply the "correct" answers through their questions. They may not have the patience to allow the quiet, to allow the chance for opening and release and resolution of that which is stuck further below in the client's body. How we can we learn to be still and allow the patron's inner being to feel safe enough to come forth, especially when we can clearly "see" their problem?

Head to open head: While not the easiest configuration, the two partners are at least speaking the same language! This goes a long way towards creating health. But the caveat here is that quite often intuition is left at the door while science, facts, thoughts are dissected—and feelings are ignored. It may be a real struggle for an open head practitioner to move beyond that head connection and lead the head-centered patron down into their body and their feelings. When it can be accomplished, potentially very good work can happen.

Head to open heart: The "head" practitioner often has trouble relating to this open heart partner. What to do? First, keep the language anchored in feelings; encourage the expression of feelings instead of explaining to the client partner what they are feeling and why. Allow feelings! This is difficult for some caregivers, I think, because they truly haven't moved through their own bodymindcores fully and can't actually reach that heart center. Learn to accept the idea of feelings as the appropriate metaphor; work with the client to reach their feeling center. Make it all right to have those feelings, and create safety by matching the style and content of the partner. All of this goes a long way in enabling healing and release to take place. And (returning to Levine) learn to allow the patron to stay anchored in body sensations, which may be difficult for some head-centered practitioners.

Head to open gut: If it's hard for a head to coax a heart, it's harder still to get that head to coax a gut to open and respond. To me, the gut represents instinct, intuition and discernment… Too often we override the gut and engage it in judgment mode instead of discernment. A head particularly judges, while a gut should discern, given the chance. Can you see how a healing partner coming from the head will try to impose judgment on the gut instead of coaxing the gut's discernment? They are standing at the edge of the well, watching the drowning patron, and thinking about which tool might be most effective, or even lecturing them about how to swim. Meanwhile, the patron may be drowning.

Head to open groin: Now it gets personal for all of us. Even more than when we talked to the groin earlier, this becomes the place to really dissect the difficulties we have with groins…by relating groin to head. I tend to agree with Reich's interpretation that too many of us are blocking our groin energy. I previously shared the idea that orgasmic energy is *not* dependent on orgasm; it's simply energy that orgasm helps to move through the body. Like a good flush through a clogged drainpipe, the orgasm releases stuck energy. Like reconnecting two electrical wires so the lights can all come on, energy that was blocked can now move again. Can we learn that stuck energy can be released without physical orgasm, if we concentrate on simply moving energy through the body, touching it, feeling it and living in it, in all aspects and locations, psychically as well as physically?

If the orgasmic energy can't rise through the groin, how can it nurture gut, heart or head? Often we ignore or suppress the groin and move higher up the chain, usually to the head, and get trapped. Sometimes we remain trapped in an underactive groin, where it languishes while a more superficial nervous energy seems to activate and operate the rest of the bodymindcore, living either in the head, or perhaps in the gut or heart. Someone who appears to operate from the head (either of the healing partners) may well be hiding from feeling their groin.

Too often these bodymindcore blocks are at the root of health challenges. The Franks see a lack of caring and validation from the outer world; Porges and Levine see a lack of the feeling of safety. Hay and Schutz sense the lack of self-esteem. Moore suggests disease is based on lack of soul awareness, while Reich and Pierrakos focus on the lack of orgasmic or core energy. Steenkamp sees in most of us a lack of courage to look deeply within, and I see a lack of bodymindcore transmission and integrity in too many of us. These are the lacks that create illness instead of wellbeing, turning "live" backwards, into "evil," into hell. All models are based in that discovery or remembrance of how to reactivate the flow of energy and restore or re-morale-ize the ability that maintains that flow.

How will it be possible for one head-centered practitioner who hides their groin, to talk to another head partner who is hiding their groin, and do any meaningful work? Two heads, ignoring the problems in both groins...can the most productive work be accomplished with this configuration? Shouldn't the practitioner partner be able to admit their own energetic block of groin, know they are living in their head as a result, and lovingly, ethically, with awareness of boundaries and fears, challenge that other head into the lower body? And again, if the self core work in the practitioner hasn't yet been done, to examine and own personal energetic problems in the groin, can we trust ourselves enough to work with others' personal energetic groin issues? Or should we send them to someone else? Can we have the courage to do the healing work of moving orgasmic energy (without sexual release being involved) on any one level at the expense of the level that really needs the work? If we can, the potential to help such a patron is great.

In my experience many people who live primarily in their heads do so because of some early sexual or emotional abuse that taught them to retreat to their "safe" room. "I'll just hide at the top of the tree until the danger goes away, then I'll climb back down a bit..." Yet the danger is no longer named, or possibly even remembered, and still they hide at the top of the tree. As practitioners, these are the very people who have the potential to sort out their own issues that keep them from grounding—and then provide very real help to others who have been through similar processes and learned to live in *their* heads, blocking *their* feelings from the rest of *their* bodies.

Before we consider a practitioner with a closed head center, let's notice someone who *doesn't use their head at all*. Perhaps they don't even live *in* their body. They're out there. They don't have clarity in their head center. They're the massage therapists who have two clients a week and charge very little for their work. They're the egoic "I-can-fix-everything-about-you and don't look at my life" practitioners. They're the people who give two and three hours of undivided attention and undercharge in too many cases. They're the ones whose stomachs are still so tied in knots that they can't get out of their groins, or hearts. They're not sure where they live in their body; perhaps outside of it. They're the ones a friend once self-described as being "heavenly minded and no earthly good." We might call them dissociated, or even schizophrenic. We could definitely call them ungrounded. Have they done their work before working with others?

One of the more effective combinations of practitioner head to patron gut is the closed head center of the practitioner as it relates to the open gut of the patron. If the practitioner doesn't normally operate from their own head, they have a "head" start in getting down to the lower center issues. Potentially they can deal with a closed groin because the two may well meet in the gut or heart region. Likewise with either an open heart or head patron, a practitioner who isn't in their head may be able to locate the active center in the patron and communicate from their own and with the patron's center.

Like so many other combinations, a closed head practitioner who relates to an open groin patron may find trouble fairly quickly. If they're already anchored below their head and the patron offers energy from the groin, it may be hard to resist the urge to "heal" that patron. Other tricky combinations for a closed head practitioner are the closed gut and the closed heart... If either of these two configurations occurs, it suggests that either the patron lives in their head, making things safer for the practitioner, or the patron moves into lower energy centers of gut and groin. Here again, caution must be used.

Let's add in one physical concept for this chapter, designed to further open the hourglass between heart and head. As you sit in your chair, move forward, away from its back. Put both hands on the back of your head, just at the top. Now, pull your chin to your chest while you ask the back of your neck both to lengthen and to arc backward. Try to create a longer and fuller curve in the back of the neck. Hold this position for several breaths; then check to see if your mind seems a bit clearer. Did you bring energy between heart and head? This is a great stop anytime and anywhere exercise that restores energy to the head with just a few seconds' work. (Remember, you'll find four awareness exercises for the four centers in Appendix A.)

And remember, this model is my current line of thought and a work in progress. If it challenges you, I invite you to visit Tables 1–8 in Appendix B and see where you agree or disagree. Can we begin to allow the realization that we do block and we do overuse certain parts of our being? Recognizing this truth is the first step toward changing it.

I'm reminded that many schools of thought teach that our greatest strengths are usually also our greatest weaknesses. Depending on which side of the coin you choose, stubbornness may be seen as tenacity; or perfectionism may be seen as organization. This is true for the use of any particular center of the body from which we tend to operate—we can make any characteristic a strength or weakness, depending on our awareness. I'd like to see more of us as practitioners learn to use all four of these centers in our work.

I *believe* it's possible to recognize (and honor) the center of the body one primarily uses; then to gear one's work toward honoring that center and modifying its effect, depending on the patron who shows up and their needs. I *think* if we allow ourselves to begin using this model, we'll be better equipped to begin allowing our personal elevator to stop on all floors. I *feel* it's important to challenge us as helpers to think in this model. It's yet another worthwhile tool for helping us get better at getting people better. I *know* most of us who do this work want to communicate to each center better, in order to help others to be better. When we're better able to match the client's centers to our own, we more fully, respectfully and caringly reach them, create safety for them, and provide for them that validating and non-judging space which is so important for healing and health.

CHAPTER 13

THE HOLY WHOLE HELPER

NEXT LAYER

The pace on the journey to healing can only be set by the client.
Jo Steenkamp[1]

...we become better helpers if and when we can suspend judgment
of patrons while discerning honestly who and where we are.
Noah Karrasch

By this time you've been inundated by my belief in doing one's own work before deciding to interfere with the situations of others. Let me disclaim once more: I haven't arrived yet! I'm still in process, the same as all of us still on the planet. What I do believe is that the longer I work with the principles of providing caring, creating safety, explaining what I do and why, and asking for participation and enthusiasm from the patron, and as I remember to consider where in their body my patron lives and how I can best reach them to interact, the better my results as a "healer" seem to be.

So, what do I mean by the "holy whole" helper of this chapter's title? In my model, this holy whole helper is one who can rise through the four centers I've discussed throughout this book. They can live in groin, gut, heart and head and operate from any of those centers as required to match, challenge and coax the patron's centers to activate or soften so as to resolve trauma or unprocessed information. If truly healthy, they're also able to operate from what might be called the seventh or crown chakra, what I prefer to think of as the "higher self." This higher self can be thought of not just in terms of what's best for *me* (the lower body, the I/me ego), but what's best for *us* (the I/you/we) when I work with *you*.

In addition, the holy whole helper can maintain a strong connection to that first chakra survival center which keeps him or her from being destroyed by sympathy for others, while staying in touch with that higher power at the same time. So I see all centers as governed by the upper, higher power *if and when we clear the lower blocks* to give the higher center its power. For those of us trapped in a lower center, this is difficult! How do we move to the higher self when we've been trapped in the gut for most of our life? How do we get the emotional elevator to operate happily from survival, through satisfaction, to self-esteem, purpose, clarity and caring health work from the highest source?

In previous chapters I have briefly described my belief in the importance of our diaphragm muscle. I've explained my model of the diaphragm acting as a primary stricture of the body, between upper (head and heart) and lower (gut and groin). Many of the combinations illustrated in previous chapters deal with the fact that too many of us have trouble moving between upper and lower body centers. This diaphragmatic hourglass controls the breath which is so important to health. Suddenly, we're back to the beginning of the book and the importance of breath. A resilient diaphragm allows energy to flow between upper and lower centers more easily, and the free flow of breath enhances this resilience in the diaphragm and gives energy to the entire body elevator.

If you allow yourself to think and feel in this head/heart/gut/groin model, chances are you already know of patrons, and of friends and family members (and yourself, if you're honest), whom you see as anchored in a particular body center. Perhaps it's your wide-hipped Granny who is stuck in the groin center and probably never appreciated sex, or your painfully thin and shy niece whose stomach is tied in knots. Maybe you have a too-loving cousin who continues to give his heart away only to have it broken again; or a too-intellectual brother who can explain anything you might want to know, but never seems to feel or even care what you're talking about. Maybe you know someone who's "heavenly minded, but no earthly good," or someone who is both promiscuous but fragile at the same time. We see all these people, all the time, if we only look.

So my point not only in this chapter, but throughout the book is that we become better helpers if and when we suspend judgment of patrons, while discerning honestly who and where *we* are. We need to admit that some of the slowed-down energetic congestion patrons show us is our own, instead of assigning the entire problem to the patron. Then we can create a safe space for them and inspire them to assume responsibility for their own healing, while keeping our own ego centers from contributing confusion to the blocks or overactivity in theirs.

I have talked about my belief in touching the appropriate layer. There's always another layer to be explored, released and hopefully resolved! As I suggested earlier in this book, unless one has ascended, one probably has more work to do on the self. It's an ongoing process, this unwinding of the bodymindcore and its traumas, and too many of us decide to stop very early in the journey. One of the joys of my nearly 30 years' career in bodywork is the enthusiasm I still find for learning new things and (I hope) improving both myself and my techniques.

So, besides doing our own work, how do we become better helpers? Foremost, we must not judge our patrons. Judgment stops our energy, and theirs. If we knew or understood their path and their process, we could come to the realization that they've coped as best they knew how in the circumstances. If we were to walk in their shoes, we might know a bit more about the whys of the path they've taken, and understand how they've arrived at the unintended destination they've reached. Not one of us got out of bed and said to self: "I'm going to really screw up my world and my life today, just for the sheer joy of it." Too many are trapped in the past, the mistakes of the past, and the fears we experienced as we made mistakes in the past or realized the consequences of our mistakes. This burdensome past that creates a fearful future is what we all want and need help in changing, moving through and resolving. Patient healing requires us to have the mindset that we offer what we have, we leave our prescriptions at the door, and we empathize and create space for unhealthy, blocked energy finally to be examined and expressed on its way to being

released and resolved. (By the way, this last sentence could be given as one definition of caring.)

Second, having chosen to be a neutral advocate for the patron, we create that space of safety that allows them to open, reveal and remove that which no longer serves them. We move energy when we invite opening. Opening may look like picking at old wounds. It may look like wanting to run from the process. It's often painful, but if we can keep patrons this side of fighting, or fleeing, or freezing, we help them feel and heal. We find ways to keep them in their process, in their discomfort and in their fear, while they learn to breathe, stretch, examine and dissolve what they *feel*. We teach them to find and feel safety, and coax them to restore resilience. *And if we don't challenge ourselves, then we shouldn't be doing it to others.*

Explaining who we are, what we do, and why we do it goes a long way toward getting the patron to come aboard. When we're aware of the head/heart/gut/groin emotional center model, we understand from where we tend to operate our own machinery, and where the patron tends to center or hide their own energy. Then we can begin to help patrons move out of and through that stuck or overused center, out of that old, unresolved thought form, out of that dis-ease or dis-order that was long ago created, and perhaps saved their life, but is no longer useful or necessary. We don't need to explain the entire head/heart/gut/groin model to every patron; but it is helpful to be better at communicating with them who you are, what you do and why.

Equally important: getting the patron onboard! "This is what I'm doing with you, this is why I'm doing it, this is what you might feel, and *this is how I need you to help me help you.*" When you can clearly communicate these ideas to your patron, you stand a much better chance of helping them make the changes they truly want to make. When a patron understands the "why" of a model, and believes it has value, energy has already been enhanced. We all want to be better; we just need help. If indeed you're a helper, you want your patrons to achieve that state of "better," but you realize they must find it for themselves. If "better" comes through you specifically and singularly and without their participation, you've robbed them of their power,

their will, and ultimately taken something important from them. You've neither released nor resolved problems, and you've not created the resilience that helps them find health.

Last, as well as first, and perhaps most important: As we get the patron onboard, let's remember their process is about them! I urge us all to remember to be aware of our own faults, frailties, blocks and challenges and to make sure we're not filtering our patrons' lives and processes and problems through our own dirty filter. Let's not make patrons sick to our standards so as to enhance our self-worth and our belief in our own healing abilities. Let's honestly examine who we are before discerning who they are and what we might or might not be able to give them. Let's heal self, or at least seek healing of self, instead of trying to heal self through others. Simple, not easy. Always, it comes back to energy and its flow or lack. If you're not doing everything in your power to keep energy flowing in and through every fiber of your being, you might not be the most effective healing partner you could be...for your spouse, your child, your coworker, your patron/client/patient or anyone else you encounter.

And keep in mind the words "release" and "resolve." Which are we attempting? While helping someone to release their pains and anxieties may be useful, doesn't resolving them sound more productive? We can remain in a world where we invite people to come to us and come back to us as we release symptoms, or we can challenge them, and ourselves, to get better at resolving the root issue instead just releasing its symptoms.

Remember this book is written from the perspective of a bodyworker; not a scientist, and certainly not a doctor or psychologist. I suggest one last time that both science and intuition are important and we shouldn't rely on only one wheel of the bicycle. I think the truths I'm trying to unearth serve us all, regardless of the path we've chosen to walk in our quest to help others find healing. And from a bodywork perspective, I'm now going to try to summarize everything I want to say in one paragraph, in words that I hope will reach all of us who want to help others, so that we can become more effective in the work we do, and perhaps even earn that label of healer, whether we want it or don't. So, my concluding thoughts:

When clients or patrons or patients understand that we're caringly creating a non-judging setting of safety so they can unwind, and when we explain what we're doing and how they can help, and when we get them on board in their own process, magic can happen. If we'll pay attention to our own process we'll realize each patron who crosses our path has a mirror piece of our own woundedness, and is there to help us heal as well. The more courageously we look at our own wounds, the more compassion and the less judgment we have for the person who presents to us. The more fully we care about the wounds that capture their energy and that they want to heal, the more they feel our caring and trust our intention. Our job is to empower them in their quest to let energy flow through their being and into our universe.

So see this book as a challenge to you, the "healer," the helper, the caregiver, the practitioner partner. Challenge yourself to find and feel your own feelings, all through your body, instead of allowing self to fight, or flee, or freeze. Challenge your patrons to use the permission to feel that you give them through your honesty, your non-judgmental attitude, your validation of their being. Challenge your model of healing, your assumptions, your belief that you have it all sorted out before the patron comes through the door. Give your best in every moment, to every patron, to every relationship.

Be blessed, live fully, and enjoy your creation of effective therapeutic relationships as you travel your path.

APPENDIX A

FOUR AWARENESS EXERCISES TO BRING ENERGY TO GROIN, GUT, HEART AND HEAD

GROIN

Lie on the floor or a bed, on your back. Extend first one heel and straight leg as far away from the hip as possible, while jamming the other heel *with a straight leg* as close as you can toward the tailbone. Then extend the tightened leg/heel, pressing the formerly lengthened heel and straight leg as close as you can to your tailbone. Next, focus on keeping the low back down into the floor as you extend the heel, while breathing and putting awareness into your pelvic floor and low belly. Can you allow yourself to find the pelvic area and feel energy stirring there? Too many of us are afraid of what we might find, and so don't allow any flow in the pelvis.

GUT

Lie on the floor, press your fingertips into your low belly just above the pubic bone, and gently and slowly drag them, fairly deeply, up the front of your spine, through your stomach, and toward your ribcage and costal arch. Intend to bring lower body energy higher in the body. Stay present and breathe deeply. Feel the rise of energy and the feelings in your groin that emanate from that rise of energy. Allow those feelings to be good feelings, and allow yourself to enjoy those good feelings throughout your body. Go slowly, experiment with allowing both breath and awareness to rise with your fingers. As you gently proceed through the stomach, stop and experience the feelings you usually hold inside your gut or groin.

HEART

Roll up a towel, or place a pillow on the floor, and lie on it with the bolster or pillow at about the tenth rib, or halfway up your spine— the bottom of your most forward curving part of spine. Bring your chin toward your chest while the back of your neck stays long. Focus literally on "opening your heart" by trying to pop open a too-shortened front of spine in the heart hinge area. As you breathe, work to visualize the front of your body around the heart getting more open, freer and energized. Can you move energy to the heart? Think of so many of our daily activities: computing, sitting, driving, detail work. Realize how much time we spend pushing ourselves into a fetal position and closing our own "heart hinge" which stops the energetic flow between gut and heart.

HEAD

As you sit in your chair, move forward, away from its back. Put both hands on the back of your head, just at the top. Now, pull your chin to your chest while you ask the back of your neck both to lengthen and to arc backward. Try to create a longer and fuller curve in the back of the neck. Hold this position for several breaths; then check to see if your mind seems a bit clearer. Did you bring energy between heart and head? This is a great stop anytime and anywhere exercise that restores energy to the head with just a few seconds' work.

APPENDIX B

TABLES OF OPEN AND CLOSED PRACTITIONER CENTERS AS THEY RELATE TO OPEN AND CLOSED PATRON CENTERS

TABLE 1: OPEN GROIN PRACTITIONER RELATING TO VARIOUS PATRONS

Center	State	Potential	Notes on Relationship
Groin	O	5	Open Groin Patron: This combination is a disaster waiting to happen! When both patron and practitioner live in overactive or open groin energy, one or the other may "accidentally" initiate behavior in a desire to move energy.
	C	4	Closed Groin Patron: Even when the groin energy of the patron is closed, an unscrupulous practitioner may try to "coax" energy into the groin area of the patron to help "heal" them.
Gut	O	4	Open Gut Patron: This patron is already grounded and doesn't live in their head. They are easy prey for an unscrupulous practitioner whose energy is centered in their groin. Still a dangerous combination.
	C	3	Closed Gut Patron: This patron, probably living higher in the body, is less likely to be pulled into the energy of an open practitioner groin, but still may be pulled into their blocked energy center. While one of the more safe combinations, still one where one needs to tread carefully.
Heart	O	4	Open Heart Patron: Still a potential disaster! A patron whose energy emanates primarily from the heart is a likely candidate to be pulled into a practitioner's groin energy, and said practitioner may pull.
	C	4	Closed Heart Patron: Still a likely problem…even with a closed heart center (unless they live totally in the head), a patron is susceptible to the groin energy of a practitioner who can claim to be an authority and offer service.
Head	O	3	Open Head Patron: A practitioner with groin issues may even be able to coax a head-centered patron to "heal" groin issues. Care must be used in this as well as all groin issues.
	C	4	Closed Head Patron: A patron living primarily from their heart center or anywhere below is still a prime candidate for abuse by a groin-centered practitioner. Remember, if a practitioner's groin is overactive, no patron is or can feel safe!

O=Open center C=Closed center 1=excellent changes possible 5=dangerous situation

TABLE 2: CLOSED GROIN PRACTITIONER RELATING TO VARIOUS PATRONS

Center	State	Potential	Notes on Relationship
Groin	O	4	Open Groin Patron: Will flirt and demand attention, and try to engage the practitioner inappropriately. If the practitioner is blocked in their own groin and living higher up, probably in the head, hopefully there will be no inappropriate intersection. They may be challenged!
	C	3	Closed Groin Patron: Both patron and practitioner will tend to live in or near their heads and possibly hearts in this scenario; therefore there is less likelihood of inappropriate behavior but also less chance of meaningful work being done.
Gut	O	2	Open Gut Patron: This patron tends to have a sense of discernment, and with the closed groin of the practitioner, they very well may be able to meet in the middle of the body and accomplish real change.
	C	3	Closed Gut Patron: If the practitioner is closed in groin and the patron in gut, chances are both are living in the head center. While they therefore communicate well, again the chances of meaningful change at the gut-level are diminished.
Heart	O	3	Open Heart Patron: While there's less chance of any kind of sexually inappropriate behavior with this combination, again, less is accomplished when the patron lives in the heart and the practitioner lives in the head...this is the challenge for the practitioner.
	C	3	Closed Heart Patron: Where do they live instead? If in the groin, trouble can ensue. If in the head, same as above: it becomes harder to make real changes if the patron and practitioner both are locked at the top of the system.
Head	O	3	Open Head Patron: While some good dialog may happen, is it meaningful dialog if both are in the head and ignoring the body? Remember, Levine suggests keeping patrons anchored in bodies.
	C	2	Closed Head Patron: If patron lives below head and practitioner lives above groin, they have a better chance of meeting somewhere in the middle, either in gut or heart space. There is the potential for real progress to happen between these two.

O=Open center C=Closed center 1=excellent changes possible 5=dangerous situation

TABLE 3: OPEN GUT PRACTITIONER RELATING TO VARIOUS PATRONS

Center	State	Potential	Notes on Relationship
Groin	O	4	Open Groin Patron: This is still too close to the groin area for comfort; it's possible this patron can coax the practitioner, with suggestive behavior, to enter their overactive groin area and participate.
	C	3	Closed Groin Patron: This has potential to be a good combination: If the patron is not in their gut, chances are they're living higher in the body, possibly heart but probably head. Can practitioner ground them further down in their body with gut energy?
Gut	O	1	Open Gut Patron: Potentially one of the best combinations. If two people can meet in gut-level honesty and remain in discernment instead of judgment, good things can happen for both, particularly for the patron.
	C	3	Closed Gut Patron: This is a frustrating situation for both… If practitioner is open and patron is closed in the gut, they'll have a harder experience trying to find common ground. Patron will tend to be judgmental while practitioner is trying to discern.
Heart	O	1	Open Heart Patron: This can be a useful and productive pairing. When practitioner with an open and discerning gut can connect with a safe and open heart through the diaphragm stricture, good work is accomplished.
	C	2	Closed Heart Patron: This can still be a useful combination. Though if the patron is in the groin, the above caveats apply; chances are they live in the head, however. If so, perhaps the two will learn to meet in the heart center, where excellent work can be done.
Head	O	3	Open Head Patron: Though in the previous line we suggest this combination can work, it's a bit difficult to get a head to talk to a gut. A sophisticated and aware practitioner can make this a very good combination, however.
	C	2	Closed Head Patron: This suggests if the head center is closed, the patron already lives in one of the lower three… If this is correct, chances are good it's heart or head, and there is room for real progress in the relationship.

O=Open center C=Closed center 1=excellent changes possible 5=dangerous situation

TABLE 4: CLOSED GUT PRACTITIONER RELATING TO VARIOUS PATRONS

Center	State	Potential	Notes on Relationship
Groin	O	4	Open Groin Patron: It's still hard to convince an open groin patron to let go of their inappropriate need to be loved, which is too often translated into sexual energy. A closed gut may suggest a jump into practitioner groin to join the patron.
	C	3	Closed Groin Patron: Safer than an open groin patron, but still can be a difficult situation. Assume the practitioner lives in heart or head; a goal may be to bring patron into their groin, safely. Risky work.
Gut	O	4	Open Gut Patron: This patron truly will go in any direction, so will follow the lead of the practitioner. Warning to practitioner therefore, to know where they want to lead this patron and use extreme caution.
	C	3	Closed Gut Patron: Chances are this patron, like the practitioner, is living in either head or heart. Where are the two? If both in head, both judge… If both in heart, both feel. If one in each place, it's harder to communicate. Practitioner responsibility to move.
Heart	O	2	Open Heart Patron: A practitioner blocked at the gut has a more difficult time sharing discernment as they can't feel it…can tend to judge. However, the open heart of the patron often can overcome the blocks of the practitioner!
	C	3	Closed Heart Patron: If the patron's heart center is closed and the practitioner's gut is closed, they may have a difficult time with basic communication, not understanding how to frame messages or requests.
Head	O	3	Open Head Patron: Where does the practitioner live? If they're closed in the gut, they may be in the heart instead; this is a tricky door to try to open between head and heart. If they live in the head as well, again, both judge and neither discerns.
	C	2	Closed Head Patron: This can actually be a better space if the practitioner is in either head or heart…they can challenge the patron to both use their head and move between areas. Downside is they don't live well in their own discernment.

O=Open center C=Closed center 1=excellent changes possible 5=dangerous situation

TABLE 5: OPEN HEART PRACTITIONER RELATING TO VARIOUS PATRONS

Center	State	Potential	Notes on Relationship
Groin	O	4	Open Groin Patron: This patron will continue to search for intimacy; a practitioner with an open heart may be pulled into the drama and neediness of such a patron. Extreme caution is needed with this partner.
	C	3	Closed Groin Patron: A heart-centered practitioner may choose to try too hard to help a closed groin patron reach their sexual feelings; still a recipe for disaster, though not as tricky as an open groin patron.
Gut	O	2	Open Gut Patron: Potential for some good work here! If the patron is open in the discernment area, and the practitioner has heart energy, they may be able to meet through the diaphragm restriction. Well worth pursuing.
	C	3	Closed Gut Patron: Where does the patron live instead? If they're in the groin, this is a tricky combination; likewise in the head. A heart to heart can be satisfactory, as can the other two combinations, with caution.
Heart	O	2	Open Heart Patron: Potential for some of the best work; the true "heart-to-heart" confrontation of issues, with the safety of sensing practitioner coming from their heart space as well. Warning: these two can become "soul mates," crossing boundaries.
	C	3	Closed Heart Patron: Again, if they're living above it may be possible to bring that patron down into heart space. If they're in gut or groin, potential for misunderstandings can occur.
Head	O	3	Open Head Patron: An aware practitioner will recognize their differences and change their language from feelings language to rational words, creating the space to invite the head patron to live more fully in the heart and lower.
	C	2	Closed Head Patron: If patron doesn't live in head, chances are good they may be in either gut or heart; either is reachable by an open heart practitioner. Again, if patron is stuck in groin, problems may arise for an open heart practitioner.

O=Open center C=Closed center 1=excellent changes possible 5=dangerous situation

TABLE 6: CLOSED HEART PRACTITIONER RELATING TO VARIOUS PATRONS

Center	State	Potential	Notes on Relationship
Groin	O	3	Open Groin Patron: Caution, as always with an open groin patron. Does the practitioner live more above or below the heart? Above, should be no problem, below may create a problem.
	C	4	Closed Groin Patron: If a patron's groin is closed and a practitioner's heart is closed, these are two of the most difficult spots to exchange information through when both are impaired. Where do both people live instead?
Gut	O	2	Open Gut Patron: Potential for a very good relationship… chances are the practitioner lives in either gut (very good) or head (can still be a good relationship). Work of practitioner is to find common ground, again.
	C	3	Closed Gut Patron: Mixed bag…a head practitioner may find the closed gut patron above the gut, a gut practitioner may be very frustrated by relationship. Either works to enhance discernment of a possibly judgmental patron.
Heart	O	4	Open Heart Patron: When the patron wants to "pour their heart out" and the practitioner believes in keeping the heart closed, it will be difficult to establish the rhythm necessary to allow resolution for the patron.
	C	3	Closed Heart Patron: Again: Where do they live instead? A closed heart practitioner and a closed heart patron may meet somewhere else in the body, or may be far apart in the body. Either way, it's difficult to have a "heart to heart."
Head	O	2	Open Head Patron: Chances are good a closed heart practitioner will live in the head. This implies a good chance for connection. Warning: can the relationship move out of the head into the rest of the body?
	C	3	Closed Head Patron: If patron is closed head and practitioner is closed heart, where will they meet? If both are anchored in the gut, good work can happen. However, often this pairing will frustrate both.

O=Open center C=Closed center 1=excellent changes possible 5=dangerous situation

TABLE 7: OPEN HEAD PRACTITIONER RELATING TO VARIOUS PATRONS

Center	State	Potential	Notes on Relationship
Groin	O	2	Open Groin Patron: One of the safest places to work from when dealing with an open groin patron; usually difficult to bring a head practitioner into a groin's issues. Heart and gut will interfere before problems arise.
	C	2	Closed Groin Patron: Again, whether open or closed in groin, if issues of groin arise, a head practitioner may be a safe and effective partner. Possible communication problems if patron lives in heart or gut, and if in head, may not get to real issues.
Gut	O	4	Open Gut Patron: Very difficult to get a gut patron to communicate with a head practitioner; two very disparate styles! If head can realize they must ground theories for patron, work is possible.
	C	3	Closed Gut Patron: Actually a better chance to work with a closed gut than an open one; if patron is stuck in groin a head may talk them through it; if patron is stuck in heart or head, still a reasonable chance to make progress.
Heart	O	3	Open Heart Patron: A head and heart always have challenges trying to communicate in each other's language. This permutation can work, but can the practitioner remember to keep the work in feeling language instead of theories?
	C	3	Closed Heart Patron: This can be a frustrating patron for an open head, or a very rewarding one… If they both live in head, lots of words fly; if patron lives in gut, responsibility on practitioner to meet them there.
Head	O	2	Open Head Patron: When both patron and practitioner live in their heads, they clearly match styles easily and the patron feels trust. Difficulty arises when "head" practitioner tries to access the patron's feelings.
	C	3	Closed Head Patron: Where do they live? Chances are the practitioner "head" will have to try to find and match that level. How skilled are they at leaving their comfortable head space to match?

O=Open center C=Closed center 1=excellent changes possible 5=dangerous situation

TABLE 8: CLOSED HEAD PRACTITIONER RELATING TO VARIOUS PATRONS

Center	State	Potential	Notes on Relationship
Groin	O	4	Open Groin Patron: If practitioner head is closed, they're living most likely in heart, then gut, then groin... Any of these three threatens to bring practitioner down into groin issues of patron. Caution here.
	C	2	Closed Groin Patron: Whether working to release groin energy or other issues, if patron lives above and practitioner is somewhere in the middle, they have a better chance of meeting and resolving instead of talking past each other.
Gut	O	2	Open Gut Patron: If the practitioner's head is closed they're likely in heart/gut; if this is the case, things are in place for gut-level honesty. Potentially one of the more effective situations.
	C	4	Closed Gut Patron: Very hard to predict where this goes: A closed head practitioner and a closed gut patron may meet in the heart, which will often be quite effective; yet it's entirely possible they're both tied to groin issues just as easily.
Heart	O	2	Open Heart Patron: This can be a good combination: If the practitioner doesn't live in their head, they're usually in gut or groin and either of these will be an effective place from which to work with the open heart patron.
	C	3	Closed Heart Patron: Where do they meet? Probably it won't be heart or head; can they meet in the gut without getting stuck in groin issues? All being well, a closed head practitioner has an open heart and can coax the closed heart patron to open.
Head	O	2	Open Head Patron: When both patron and practitioner live in their heads, they clearly match styles easily and the patron feels trust. Difficulty arises when "head" practitioner tries to access patron feelings.
	C	2	Closed Head Patron: Clearly, if both heads are closed, the pair will meet somewhere below. Unless this meeting is in the groin, they will be able to resolve at the heart and gut-level, where true work occurs.

O=Open center C=Closed center 1=excellent changes possible 5=dangerous situation

REFERENCES

PROLOGUE

1. Smith, S. (1988) *4T's for Tithing of Time, Talent, and Treasure.* Lees Summit, MO: Unity School of Christianity. Available at www.4Tprosperity.com, accessed on 4 June 2014.

2. Lupton, D. (2012) *Medicine as Culture: Illness, Disease and the Body* (3rd ed.). London, Thousand Oaks, CA, New Delhi: Sage Publications. pp.viii, ix.

3. Karrasch, N. (2009) *Meet Your Body: CORE Bodywork and Rolfing Tools to Release Bodymindcore Trauma.* London and Philadelphia: Singing Dragon.

4. Karrasch, N. (2012) *Freeing Emotions and Energy Through Myofascial Release.* London and Philadelphia: Singing Dragon.

CHAPTER 1

1. Porges, S. *The Polyvagal Theory for Treating Trauma.* Interview with Dr. Ruth Buczynski. Available at http://stephenporges.com/index.php/component/content/article/5-popular-articles/25-nicabm-the-polyvagal-theory-for-treating-trauma, accessed on 4 June 2014. Reprinted by permission of Stephen Porges.

2. See http://medical-dictionary.thefreedictionary.com/defensive+medicine, accessed on 4 June 2014.

3. Brill, S. (2013) "Why medical bills are killing us." *Time Magazine.* 4 March.

4. Moore, T. (2010) *Care of the Soul in Medicine.* Carlsbad, CA and London: Hay House. p.158.

5. Painter, J. (1987) *Deep Bodywork and Personal Development.* Mill Valley, CA: Bodymind Books. p.164.

6. Berceli, D. (2008) *The Revolutionary Trauma Release Process: Transcend Your Toughest Times.* Vancouver, BC: Namaste. p.6.

7. Carlson, R. and Shield, B. (eds) (1989) *Healers on Healing.* Los Angeles, CA: Jeremy Tarcher.

8. Upledger, J. (1989) "Self-Discovery and Self-Healing." In Carlson and Shield (1989). p.70.

9. Hay, L. (1984) *You Can Heal Your Life and Heal Your Body.* Carlsbad, CA and London: Hay House.

10. Hay, L. and Schulz, M.L. (2013) *All is Well.* Carlsbad, CA and London: Hay House. p.168.

11. Sarno, J. (2006) *The Divided Mind.* London and New York: Harper.

12. Sarno (2006). pp.15–20.

13. Abrams, D., Dolor, R., Roberts, R. *et al.* (2013) "The BraveNet prospective observational study on integrative medicine treatment approaches for pain." *BMC Complementary and Alternative Medicine, 13,* 146.

CHAPTER 2

1. Haines, S. (2013) "Dissociation and the body." Available at www.stevehaines.net/wp-content/uploads/2011/10/dissociation-v8.pdf, accessed on 4 September 2014. p.8. Reprinted by permission of Steve Haines.

2. Tolle, E. (2006) *Through the Open Door (lectures)*. Available from www.soundstrue.com/eckhart-tolle, accessed on 4 June 2014. Reprinted by permission of Sounds True.

3. Hay, L. and Schulz, M.L. (2013) *All is Well*. Carlsbad, CA and London: Hay House. p.60.

4. Sarno, J. (2006) *The Divided Mind*. London, New York: Harper. pp.3–4.

5. Harvey, R., private letter. See also *The Fulcrum* (the journal of the Craniosacral Therapy Association), January 2008.

6. Levine, P. (2010) *In an Unspoken Voice*. Berkeley, CA: North Atlantic Books.

7. Levine, P. and Kline, M. (2008) *Trauma-Proofing Your Kids*. Berkeley, CA: North Atlantic Books, and Lyons, CO: ERGOS Institute Press. p.1.

8. On *Trauma Informed Care* see www.traumainformedcareproject.org, accessed on 4 June 2014.

9. Berceli, D. (2008) *The Revolutionary Trauma Release Process: Transcend Your Toughest Times*. Vancouver, BC: Namaste. pp.7, 25.

10. Orlinsky, D. and Howard, K. (1986) "Generic Model of Psychotherapy." Available at http://de.wikipedia.org/wiki/Generic_Model_of_Psychotherapy, accessed on 4 June 2014.

11. Frank, J. and Frank, J. (1961, 1991) *Persuasion and Healing*. Baltimore, MD and London: Johns Hopkins University Press.

12. Frank and Frank (1961, 1991). p.157.

13. Schutz, W. (1994) *The Human Element*. San Franscisco, CA: Jossey-Bass Publishers. p.xiii.

14. Twerski, A.J. (1990) *Addictive Thinking: Understanding Self-Deception*. San Francisco, CA: Harper/Hazelton. p.17.

15. Sarno (2006). pp.101, 103.

16. See Leonard-Segal, A. (2006) "A Rheumatologist's Experience with Psychosomatic Disorders." In Sarno (2006). pp.267–8.

17. Porges, S. "The Polyvagal Theory for Treating Trauma." Interview with Dr. Ruth Buczynski. Available at http://stephenporges.com/index.php/component/content/article/5-popular-articles/25-nicabm-the-polyvagal-theory-for-treating-trauma, accessed on 4 June 2014.

18. Sarno (2006). p.104.

19. Porges.

20. Fennessy, C. "Running Back From Hell." Available at http://m.runnersworld.com/runners-stories/running-back-from-hell?page=single, accessed on 4 June 2012.

21. Steenkamp, J. (2002) *SHIP: The Age-Old Art of Facilitating Healing*. Pretoria: JOS Publishing. pp.2, 50, 214.

22. Levine, P. (1997) *Waking the Tiger*. Berkeley, CA: North Atlantic Books.

23. Berceli Foundation website: www.bercelifoundation.org/s/1340/aff_2_interior.aspx?sid=1340&gid=1pgid=403.

24. Tolle, E. (2006) *New Earth: Awakening to Your Soul's Purpose*. New York: Plume/Penguin. pp.141, 144–5.

25. Scott Peck, M. (1983) *People of the Lie*. New York: Simon & Schuster. p.95.

26. Remen, R.N. cited in Rossmann, M. (1989) "Illness as an Opportunity for Healing." In Carlson, R. and Shield, B. (eds) *Healers on Healing*. Los Angeles, CA: Jeremy Tarcher. p.78; Northrup, C. (1994) *Women's Bodies, Women's Wisdom: The Complete Guide to Women's Health and Well-Being*. New York: Bantam Dell.

27. Hoffman, J. and Raman, S. "Communication Factors in Malpractice Cases." Available at www.rmf.harvard.edu/Clinician-Resources/Article/2012/Insight-Communication-Factors-in-Mal-Cases, accessed on 4 June 2014.

28. Levine (2010). pp.56, 68, 70.

29. Frank and Frank (1961, 1991). pp.35–6.

30. Frankl, V. (1984) *Man's Search for Meaning*. New York: Simon & Schuster.

CHAPTER 3

1. Taylor, K. (1995) *The Ethics of Caring*. Santa Cruz, CA: Hanford Mead. p.55. Reprinted by permission of Kylea Taylor.

2. Oschman, J. (2000) *Energy Medicine: The Scientific Basis*. Philadelphia, PA: Elsevier.

3. Arbesman, S. (2012/13) *The Half Life of Facts: Why Everything We Know Has an Expiration Date*. New York: Penguin/Current. p.4.

4. Gladwell, M. (2005) *Blink*. Boston, New York and London: Little Brown & Co./Back Bay Books. pp.136–7.

5. Hay, L. and Schulz, M. L. (2013) *All is Well*. Carlsbad, CA and London: Hay House. p.5.

6. Cited in Rossman, M. (1989) "Illness as an Opportunity for Healing." In Carlson, R. and Shield, B. (eds) *Healers on Healing*. Los Angeles, CA: Jeremy Tarcher. p.83.

7. Rochelle, J.R. (2009) "My Perspectives on Psychosomatic Medicine." In Sarno, J. (ed.) *The Divided Mind*. London and New York: Harper. p.284.

8. Bordoni, B. and Zanier, E. (2013) "Anatomic Connections of the Diaphragm and their effects of respiration on the body." *Journal of Multidisciplinary Healthcare*, 6. pp.281–91.

9. Moore, T. (2010) *Care of the Soul in Medicine*. Carlsbad, CA and London: Hay House, p.xx.

10. See www.aip.org/history/heisenberg/p08.htm.

11. Nelson, D. (2013) *The Mystery of Pain*. London and Philadelphia, PA: Singing Dragon. pp.144–5.

12. Reported in Feinburg, C. (2013) "The placebo phenomenon." Available at http://harvardmagazine.com/2013/01/the-placebo-phenomenon, accessed on 6 June 2014.

13. See http://well.blogs.nytimes.com/2014/07/23/acetaminophen-no-better-than-placebo-for-back-pain/?_php=true&_type=blogs&_r=0. Here is one study showing how traditional medicine is, in fact, no better at all.

14. Dunn, K. (2005) "The nocebo effect." Available at http://harvardmagazine.com/2005/05/the-nocebo-effect.html, accessed on 6 June 2014.

15. Enck, P., Benedetti, F. and Schedlowski, M. (2008) "New Insights into the Placebo and Nocebo Responses." *Neuron*, July, pp.195–206.

16. Hedley, G. (2013) *The Heart of Service.* Self-published. pp.70, 89. Available at www. gilheadley.com/hosbookinfo.php.

CHAPTER 4

1. Johnson, D.H. (1989) "Presence." In Carlson, R. and Shield, B. (eds) *Healers on Healing.* Los Angeles, CA: Jeremy Tarcher. p.133. Reprinted by permission of Jeremy P. Tarcher, an imprint of Penguin Group (USA) LLC.

2. Pierrakos, J. (2005) *CORE Energetics: Developing the Capacity to Love and Heal.* Mendicino, CA: CORE Evolution®.

3. Pierrakos, E. (1990) *The Pathwork of Self-Transformation.* New York: Bantam.

4. Painter, J. (1987) *Deep Bodywork and Personal Development.* Mill Valley, CA: Bodymind Books. p.186.

5. Levine, P. (2010) *In an Unspoken Voice.* Berkeley, CA: North Atlantic Books, and Lyons, CO: ERGOS Institute Press. pp.345, 340–50.

6. Sarno, J. (2006) *The Divided Mind.* London and New York: Harper. p.66.

7. Berceli, D. (2008) *The Revolutionary Trauma Release Process: Transcend Your Toughest Times.* Vancouver, BC: Namaste. p.39.

8. Ida Rolf cited by Emmett Hutchins (author's personal notes from Rolf training 1986).

9. Steenkamp, J. (2002) *SHIP: The Age-Old Art of Facilitating Healing.* Pretoria: JOS Publishing. p.18.

10. Egoscue, P. (1998) *Pain Free: A Revolutionary Method for Stopping Chronic Pain.* New York, Toronto, London, Sydney, Auckland: Bantam. p.23.

11. See www.thebodyelectricschool.com, accessed on 7 June 2014.

12. Moore, T. (2010) *Care of the Soul in Medicine.* Carlsbad, CA and London: Hay House. p.xxvi.

13. Chia, M. and Abrams, D. (1996) *The Multi-Orgasmic Man: Sexual Secrets Every Man Should Know.* San Francisco, CA: Harper. p.16.

14. Taylor, K. (1995) *The Ethics of Caring.* Santa Cruz, CA: Hanford Mead. pp.1, 3, 7, 10.

15. "Ethical Issues in Clinical Practice." Course with Sunny Cooper, 2004.

16. Pierrakos, J. (2005) *CORE Energetics: Developing the Capacity to Love and Heal.* Mendicino, CA: CORE Evolution®.

17. Brennan, B. (1988) *Hands of Light: Guide to Healing Through the Human Energy Fields.* New York, Toronto, London, Sydney, Auckland: Bantam.

18. Forni, P.N. (2002) *Choosing Civility.* New York: St Martin's Griffin.

19. Keen, L.K. *The Ethics of Touch.* Available at www.somatics.de/artikel/for-professionals/2-article/104-the-ethics-of-touch, accessed on 7 June 2014.

20. Mary Sykes Wylie cited in Taylor (1995). p.46.

CHAPTER 5

1. Levine, P. (2010) *In an Unspoken Voice.* Berkeley, CA: North Atlantic Books. p.40. Reprinted by permission of North Atlantic Books.

2. May, R. (1989) "The Empathetic Relationship: A Foundation of Healing." In Carlson, R. and Shield, B. (eds) (1989) *Healers on Healing*. Los Angeles, CA: Jeremy Tarcher. pp.108–9.

3. Steenkamp, J. (2002) *SHIP: The Age-Old Art of Facilitating Healing*. Pretoria: JOS Publishing. p.131.

4. *Healing Neen: Trauma and Recovery In the Hollow Films*. Available at http://vimeo.com/82555312, accessed on 7 June 2014.

5. Scott Peck, M. (1983/1990) *People of the Lie: The Hope for Healing Human Evil*. London: Random/Arrow. p.149.

6. Berceli, D. (2008) *The Revolutionary Trauma Release Process: Transcend Your Toughest Times*. Vancouver, BC: Namaste. p.107.

7. Grof, M.D. and Grof, C. (1989) *Spiritual Emergency: When Personal Transformation Becomes a Crisis*. Los Angeles, CA: Jeremy Tarcher.

8. Moore, T. (2010) *Care of the Soul in Medicine*. Carlsbad, CA and London: Hay House. p.165.

9. Levine (2010). p.80.

10. Levine (2010). p.35.

11. Moore (2010). p.123.

12. Kaptchuk, T. (1989) "Healing as a Journey Together." In Carlson, R. and Shield, B. (eds) *Healers on Healing*. Los Angeles, CA: Jeremy Tarcher.

13. Doucleff, M. *Mapping Emotions on the Body: Love Makes Us Warm All Over*. Available at www.npr.org/blogs/health/2013/12/30/258313116/mapping-emotions-on-the-body-love-makes-us-warm-all-over, accessed on 7 June 2014.

14. Remen, R.N. (1989) "The Search for Healing." In Carlson, R. and Shield, B. (eds) *Healers on Healing*. Los Angeles, CA: Jeremy Tarcher. p.94.

15. Chernin, D. (1985) "Holistic Medicine: Its Goals, Models, Historical Roots." In Kunz, D. (ed.) *Spiritual Aspects of the Healing Arts*. Wheaton, IL: Theosophical Publishing House. pp.102–3.

16. Schwartz, J. (1989) "Healing, Love and Empowerment." In Carlson, R. and Shield, B. (eds) *Healers on Healing*. Los Angeles, CA: Jeremy Tarcher. pp.18–20.

17. Sarno, J. (2006) *The Divided Mind*. London, New York: Harper. pp.134–5.

18. Charron, R. (2006) *Narrative Medicine: Honoring the Stories of Illness*. Oxford and New York: Oxford University Press. p.ix.

19. Gladwell, M. (2005) *Blink*. Boston, New York and London: Little Brown & Co./Back Bay Books. p.40.

20. Sanghavi, D. "Medical malpractice: Why is it so hard for doctors to apologize?" *Boston Globe Magazine*, 1 January 2013. Available at www.bostonglobe.com/magazine/2013/01/27/medical-malpractice-why-hard-for-doctors-apologize/c65KIUZraXekMZ8SHlMsQM/story.html, accessed on 4 September 2014.

21. Moore (2010). pp.10–11.

22. Sarno (2006). p.131.

23. Schwartz (1989). pp.18–20.

24. Berceli (2008). p.107.

25. Norris, P. (1989) "Healing: What We Can Learn from Children." In Carlson, R. and Shield, B. (eds) *Healers on Healing*. Los Angeles, CA: Jeremy Tarcher. p.160.

26. Taylor, K. (1995) *The Ethics of Caring*. Santa Cruz, CA: Hanford Mead. p.55.

27. Moore (2010). p.28.

28. Nelson, D. (2013) *The Mystery of Pain*. London and Philadelphia, PA: Singing Dragon. p.132.

29. Krippner, S. (1989) "Touchstones of the Healing Process." In Carlson, R. and Shield, B. (eds) *Healers on Healing*. Los Angeles, CA: Jeremy Tarcher. p.111.

30. Fay, J. and Funk, D. (1995) *Teaching with Love and Logic*. Golden, CO: Love and Logic Press. p.171.

31. Kübler-Ross, E. (1989) "The Four Pillars of Healing." In Carlson, R. and Shield, B. (eds) *Healers on Healing*. Los Angeles, CA: Jeremy Tarcher. p.127.

32. Levine (2010). pp.75–94.

CHAPTER 6

1. Moore, T. (2010) *Care of the Soul in Medicine*. Carlsbad, CA and London: Hay House. p.184. Reprinted by permission of Hay House, Inc.

2. Littlejohn, C. (2010) "The psoas: Release, or resolve?" UK Thai Magazine, June. Available at www.thaihealingalliance.com/pdf/The_Psoas,_Release_or_Resolve_-_Carmen_Littlejohn.pdf, accessed on 8 June 2014.

3. Steenkamp, J. (2002) *SHIP: The Age-Old Art of Facilitating Healing*. Pretoria: JOS Publishing. p.79.

4. Kaptchuk, T. (1989) "Healing as a Journey Together." In Carlson, R. and Shield, B. (eds) *Healers on Healing*. Los Angeles, CA: Jeremy Tarcher. p.105.

5. Hedley, G. *Integral Anatomy Series 1–4*. Video dissections. Available at www.integralanatomy.com, accessed on 8 June 2014.

6. Levine, P. (2010) *In an Unspoken Voice*. Berkeley, CA: North Atlantic Books. p.159.

7. Levine (2010). p.110.

8. Cannon, J. (2013) "Working with Noxious People." Seminar sponsored by the Institute for Brain Potential, Haddonfield, NJ.

9. Schutz, W. (1994) *The Human Element*. San Francisco, CA: Jossey-Bass Publishers. p.24.

10. Frank, J. and Frank, J. (1961, 1991) *Persuasion and Healing*. Baltimore, MD and London: Johns Hopkins University Press. p.208.

CHAPTER 7

1. Gawain, S. (1989) "Listening to Inner Wisdom." In Carlson, R. and Shield, B. (eds) *Healers on Healing*. Los Angeles, CA: Jeremy Tarcher. p.74. Reprinted by permission of Jeremy P. Tarcher, an imprint of Penguin Group (USA) LLC.

2. Moore, T. (2010) *Care of the Soul in Medicine*. Carlsbad, CA and London: Hay House. p.12. Reprinted by permission of Hay House, Inc.

3. Moore (2010). p.176.

4. Scott Peck, M. (1983/1990) *People of the Lie: The Hope for Healing Human Evil*. London: Random/Arrow. pp.82–3.

5. Steenkamp, J. (2002) *SHIP: The Age-Old Art of Facilitating Healing*. Pretoria: JOS Publishing. p.68.

6. Painter, J. (1987) *Deep Bodywork and Personal Development*. Mill Valley, CA: Bodymind Books. p.17.

7. Moore (2010). p.190.

8. Moore (2010). pp.62–3.

9. Frank, J. and Frank, J. (1961, 1991) *Persuasion and Healing*. Baltimore, MD and London: Johns Hopkins University Press. pp.165–6.

10. Painter (1987). p.17.

11. Steenkamp (2002). pp.133, 140.

CHAPTER 8

1. Moore, T. (2010) *Care of the Soul in Medicine*. Carlsbad, CA and London: Hay House. p.150. Reprinted by permission of Hay House, Inc.

2. William Shakespeare, *Hamlet*, Act II, Scene 2.

3. Karrasch, N. (2012) *Freeing Emotions and Energy Through Myofascial Release*. London and Philadelphia, PA: Singing Dragon.

4. Hay, L. and Schulz, M.L. (2013) *All is Well*. Carlsbad, CA and London: Hay House. pp.31–2.

5. Berceli, D. (2008) *The Revolutionary Trauma Release Process: Transcend Your Toughest Times*. Vancouver, BC: Namaste. p.11.

6. Levine, P. (2010) *In an Unspoken Voice*. Berkeley, CA: North Atlantic Books. p.9.

7. Agneessens, C.A. (2008) "Exploring the Use of Language in the Art of Rolfing." (Lecture transcript.)

CHAPTER 9

1. Taylor. K. (1995) *The Ethics of Caring*. Santa Cruz, CA: Hanford Mead. p.100. Reprinted by permission of Kylea Taylor.

2. Chia, M. and Abrams, D. (1996) *The Multi-Orgasmic Man: Sexual Secrets Every Man Should Know*. San Francisco, CA: Harper. p.8. Reprinted by permission of HarperCollins Publishers.

3. Hay, L. and Schulz, M.L. (2013) *All is Well*. Carlsbad, CA and London: Hay House. pp.55–6.

4. Tolle, E. (2006) *Through the Open Door*. CD. Available from www.soundstrue.com.

5. Chia and Abrams (1996). p.16.

6. Scott Peck, M. (1991) *The Road Less Travelled*. London: Arrow. pp.188–9.

7. Taylor, K. (1955) *The Ethics of Caring*. Santa Cruz, CA: Hanford Mead. p.69.

8. Taylor (1955). p.97.

CHAPTER 10

1. Matthew 7:i.

2. Scott Peck, M. (1983/1990) *People of the Lie: The Hope for Healing Human Evil*. London: Random/Arrow. p.10.

3. Gladwell, M. (2005) *Blink*. Boston, New York, and London: Little Brown & Co./Back Bay Books. p.265.

4. Berceli, D. (2008) *The Revolutionary Trauma Release Process: Transcend Your Toughest Times*. Vancouver, BC: Namaste. p.57.

5. Hay, L. and Schulz, M.L. (2013) *All is Well*. Carlsbad, CA, and London: Hay House. p.76.

6. "The Arvigo techniques of Maya Abdominal Therapy." Available at https://arvigotherapy. com, accessed on 15 June 2014.

7. Pallady, P. (2006) *Gut Instinct: What Your Stomach is Trying to Tell You*. London: Rodale International.

8. Taylor, K. (1995) *The Ethics of Caring*. Santa Cruz, CA: Hanford Mead. p.100.

CHAPTER 11

1. Tolle, E. (2006) *Through the Open Door*. CD. Available from www.soundstrue.com. Reprinted by permission of Sounds True.

2. Buckner, R. (2014) In *CORE II* newsletter (private newsletter), July. Reprinted by permission of Rod Buckner.

3. Moore, T. (2010) *Care of the Soul in Medicine*. Carlsbad, CA and London: Hay House. p.123.

4. Hay, L. and Schulz, M.L. (2013) *All is Well*. Carlsbad, CA and London: Hay House. pp.103–4.

5. Hay and Schulz (2013). p.130.

CHAPTER 12

1. Forni, P.N. (2002) *Choosing Civility*. New York: St Martin's Griffin. p.7. Reprinted by permission of Pier Forni.

2. Berceli, D. (2008) *The Revolutionary Trauma Release Process: Transcend Your Toughest Times*. Vancouver, BC: Namaste. p.134.

3. Moore, T. (2010) *Care of the Soul in Medicine*. Carlsbad, CA and London: Hay House. pp.106, 131.

4. Watts, A. (1951) *The Wisdom of Insecurity*. New York: Random House/Vintage Publishing. p.57.

5. Hay, L. and Schulz, M.L. (2013) *All is Well*. Carlsbad, CA, and London: Hay House. p.145.

CHAPTER 13

1. Steenkamp, J. (2002) *SHIP: The Age-Old Art of Facilitating Healing.* Pretoria: JOS Publishing. p.119. Reprinted by permission of Jo Steenkamp.

INDEX

Page references to footnotes will be
followed by the letter "n"

Abrams, Douglas 28, 62, 123, 126, 173n,
    176n, 179n
abuse issues 32, 165
    emotional abuse 124, 152
    sexual abuse 124, 143
acceptance 70, 82
acupuncture/acupressure 56
Addictive Thinking: Understanding Self-
    Deception (Twerski) 37, 174n
Adler, Alfred 37
adrenal system 91
afferent fibers 38
affirmations 31, 49
Alexander Technique 60
All is Well (Hay and Schulz) 25, 49, 114–
    15, 173n, 174n, 175n, 179n, 180n
allopathic medical establishment 27–8, 47
    limited communication skills 68, 81, 82
alternative medicine 47
anti-stress mechanism 38
anxiety 34–5, 83
Arbesman, Samuel 47
archetypes 63, 64, 112, 117
Arvigo therapy 138, 180n
Asian cultures 148
atmosphere of acceptance 70
attraction to therapist 129–30, 131
authority, pretending to be 101–2, 103
autonomic nervous system 39
awareness exercises 127–8, 137, 142,
    154, 163–4

balance 19, 20
Benedetti, Fabrizio 52
"benevolent regard" 65
Berceli, David 23, 34–5, 41, 42, 58, 84,
    117, 148, 149, 174n, 176n, 178n
Bible 102, 133
Bioenergetics 57

Blink (Gladwell) 49, 82, 175n, 177n, 180n
blockages
    emotional *see* emotional blockages
    groin–gut–heart–head model 17, 110,
        111, 113
    groin blockages 124, 125, 137, 158
    gut blockages 149
    heart blockages 144
    sexual/sacral (second) chakra 123–4
body armor 57
Body Electric School 61
Body of Light, The (Mann and Short) 62
body sensations 77
bodymindcore model 13, 15, 19, 24, 47,
    60, 92, 111, 150, 152
    communication skills 79, 80
    overwhelmed state 118–19
    and reasons for ill-health 34, 38, 40, 42
    restoration of energy flow 55–6
bodywork 32, 33, 40, 141
    healing models 55, 56, 60
    layering model 92–3
Bordoni, B. 50, 175n
boundaries of care 71
brain 26, 39, 52, 77, 127, 148
    gut brain 133, 149
    head brain 134
    and healing models 60, 62
    and vagus nerve 33, 38, 40, 57, 133,
        141
breath holding 23, 31, 32, 36, 44, 76,
    124
    heart-centered model 140, 141
breathing exercises/correct breathing
    32–3, 35, 38
Brennan, Barbara 64, 176n
Brill, Stephen 20
Buckner, Rod 139

Care of the Soul in Medicine (Moore) 22,
    148, 173n, 175n, 176n, 178n, 179n,
    180n

caring 67–75
  boundaries of care 71
  and empathy 68–9, 81, 91, 94, 96
  feeling cared for 52, 69, 74
  lack of care, feeling 68, 72
  non-judgmental 69, 72–3, 77, 94, 159
  settings, care work 75–7
  working together and overcoming
    difficulties 73–4
Carlson, Richard 24, 173n, 175n, 176n,
  177n, 178n
carpal tunnel problems 25, 99–100
catatonia 43
central nervous system (CNS) 39
chakra system model 56, 113–15, 121
  crown (seventh) chakra 114, 115
  heart (fourth) chakra 114
  root/survival (first) chakra 114, 115,
    127, 158
  sexual/sacral (second) chakra 114, 115,
    123–4, 127
  solar plexus (third) chakra 114
  third eye (sixth) chakra 114
  throat (fifth) chakra 114, 115, 150
Charron, Rita 80, 177n
Chernin, Dennis 79, 177n
Chia, Mantak 62, 123, 126, 176n, 179n
childhood abuse, unresolved 32
chiropractic work 59
Choosing Civility (Forni) 65, 176n, 180n
clarity safety 147–55
closed groin practitioner 113, 119, 120,
  125, 131–2, 166
closed gut practitioner 113, 119, 120,
  136, 168
closed head practitioner 113, 119, 120,
  153–4, 172
closed heart practitioner 113, 119, 120,
  170
colonic therapy 55, 56, 61
communication skills 42–3, 60, 76, 78–83
  in allopathic model 68, 81, 82
  listening 77, 79, 81
Complementary and Alternative Medicine
  (journal) 28
Comprehensive Studies program (Rolf
  Institute, Colorado) 47
concentration camps 44

congestion 20, 110, 111, 120, 124, 159
connective tissue, releasing 59
Cooper, Sunny 63, 64, 112, 117, 125
cooperation 83–7
  partnership approach to doctor–patient
    relationship 84–5
CORE Energetics (healing model) 57, 64,
  176n
CORE Fascial Release work 56, 59
counselors 56, 71, 83, 85
  emotionally unstable 101
  self-care, need for 99, 100, 103, 105
craniosacral therapy 118
crown (seventh) chakra 114, 115

death, peaceful 20
Deep Bodywork and Personal Development
  (Painter) 22–3, 58, 173n, 176n,
  179n
demoralization 36, 43, 44, 72, 111
  see also re-moral-izing of clients
diaphragm 50, 158
  hourglass stricture analogy 140–1, 143,
    149–50
Divided Mind, The (Sarno) 25
doctor–patient relationship, partnership
  approach 84–5
Dolor, R. 28, 173n

E-block 41, 71
ego 43, 58, 115, 126
  centers 110, 111, 112, 117, 159
  egotistical practitioner 102, 104, 117
Egoscue, Pete 61, 176n
embodiment 97–107
  health, failure of practitioner to embody
    98–9
E-motion (Energy in Motion) 71
emotional blockages 16, 31, 41, 43, 71
  releasing 59, 89
  see also blockages; under trauma
emotions, expressing in body 77
"empath" 68–9, 94, 145
empathy 81, 94, 96
  versus sympathy 91
Enck, Paul 52
endorphins 40

energy
　　free flow 57, 60, 61
　　　　restoration of 55–6, 62
　　gut 135, 142
　　negative 93, 95
　　orgasmic/orgone energy 57, 61, 124,
　　　　126, 127, 141, 151
　　sexual *see* sexual energy
　　slowed-down 59
　　stuck *see* stuck energy, releasing
　　universality across cultures 62
energy cyst 118
eroticism 61
ethical behavior 62–3
Ethics of Caring, The 63, 65–6, 129, 138,
　　176n
evidence-based medicine 47, 49, 50, 52,
　　148
evil 71, 101, 140
external validation 20, 69

fallibility, admitting 81, 82
fascia, releasing 59
Fay, Jim 86, 178n
feelings, allowing 150
Feldenkrais work 60
Ferreira, Valeria 22
fibers, nerve 38–9, 40
fibromyalgia 31–2, 141
fight-or-flight response 34, 38, 40, 44,
　　65, 116
"fixing" of others, erroneous belief as to
　　27, 71–2, 83, 133, 135, 153
　　healing models 53, 65
　　needs of practitioners 101, 102, 105
flexor muscles/flexor withdrawal 58
Forni, P.N. 65, 147, 176n, 180n
4T's Program (Tithing of Time, Talent and
　　Treasure) (Smith) 14
Frank, Jerome and Julia 42, 43, 66, 86,
　　87, 96, 111, 140, 144, 152, 175n,
　　178n, 179n
　　four commonalities for healing 35, 36,
　　　　67, 93
Frankl, Viktor 44, 175n
*Freeing Emotions and Energy Through
　　Myofascial Release* (Karrasch) 16, 114,
　　173n, 179n

freeze response 38, 39, 40
　　groin–gut–heart–head model 116,
　　　　118–19
Funk, David 86, 178n

Gastroesophageal Reflux Disease (GERD)
　　141
Gawain, Shakti 97, 178n
Gladwell, Malcolm 49, 82, 134, 175n,
　　177n, 180n
"goodism" (perfectionism) 25–6, 58, 154
gravity, in Rolfing technique 59
greed 28
grief 43, 72
Grof, Stan and Christina 70, 177n
groin
　　blockages 124, 125, 137, 158
　　closed groin practitioner 113, 119, 120,
　　　　125, 131–2, 166
　　open groin practitioner 113, 119, 120,
　　　　130–1, 165
　　special challenge of 17, 123
　　see also groin–gut–heart–head model
groin–gut–heart–head model 56, 62,
　　109–21
　　awareness exercises 163, 164
　　blockages 17, 110, 111, 113
　　chakra system model 113–15
　　keeping all in a straight line 16
　　see also ego; groin–gut–heart–head
　　　　model; gut; head; heart
group ethics 130
gut
　　blockages 149
　　closed gut practitioner 113, 119, 120,
　　　　136, 168
　　knots in 135, 137, 158
　　open gut practitioner 113, 119, 120,
　　　　133, 134, 135, 167
　　see also groin–gut–heart–head model
gut brain 133, 149
gut energy 135–6, 142
*Gut Instinct: What Your Stomach is Trying to
　　Tell You* (Pallardy) 138
gut-level reactions 135, 136

Haines, Steve 31
Half Life of Facts, The (Arbesman) 47

Hands of Light (Brennan) 64, 176n
Harvey, Ralph 22, 33, 38
Hay, Louise 31, 37, 42, 123, 136–7, 140, 149, 152
  All is Well 25, 49, 114–15, 173n, 174n, 175n, 179n, 180n
  Heal Your Body 25
  You Can Heal Your Life 25
head
  closed head practitioner 113, 119, 120, 153–4, 172
  living in one's head 147–8, 149
  open head practitioner 113, 119, 120, 132, 142, 149, 151, 171
  to open groin 151
  to open gut 151
  to open head 150
  to open heart 150–1
  see also groin–gut–heart–head model
Heal Your Body (Hay) 25
healer categories 63, 64, 65, 112, 117, 131
Healers on Healing (Carlson and Shield) 24, 68, 79, 84, 173n, 175n, 176n, 177n, 178n
healing 13, 14, 15, 16, 17, 43
  and balance 19, 20
  effective, four commonalities for (Frank and Frank) 35, 36, 67, 93
  healing relationship 21–2, 26, 51
  matching of technique and helper to client/patron 27
  models, choice of 55–66
  needs of practitioners 97–107, 116, 128, 161
  as ongoing process 36, 90, 98, 128
  as reciprocal act 22–3
  wounded healer 99, 102
healing mirrors 21, 26, 28, 73, 102
healing teams 28
health
  concept 21
  groin–gut–heart–head model *see* groin–gut–heart–head model
  gut 136–7
  healing models 55–66
  life choices 15–16

practitioner failing to embody 98–9
responsibility for own 15, 19, 20, 35, 69, 83, 164
  see also cooperation; participation of patron/client in therapy
working on 85
health care costs 20
heart
  closed heart practitioner 113, 119, 120, 170
  "hardened" heart, practitioner with 143, 144
  heart-centered model 139, 140
  open heart practitioner 113, 119, 120, 140, 142, 143, 169
  see also groin–gut–heart–head model
heart (fourth) chakra 114
Heart of Service, The (Hedley) 53
heart rate variability (HRV) 33, 38, 141
Hedley, Gil 53, 92, 176n, 178n
Heisenberg, Werner 50
higher self 157
Hippocratic Oath 116
holding of breath *see* breath holding
"holy whole" helper 157–62
hope 51, 71
Howard, K. 35, 36, 174n
Human Element, The (Schutz) 36–7, 95
hypnotherapy 55, 56, 60

Ida Rolf Method of Structural Integration (Rolfing) *see* Rolf, Ida/Rolfing
idols 102
illness/disorder
  airplane crash of author 13, 14, 80–1
  psychosomatic problems 25, 32, 58, 60, 109
  reasons for 31–45
In an Unspoken Voice (Levine) 33, 174n, 176n, 178n, 179n
inferiority, feelings of 37
information 24–5
  overload 49, 133
insight 47
insurance 83
internal validation 69, 73, 106

intuition 150
  placebo treatment and feeling better
    51–2, 53
  versus science 17, 47–53, 161
investment of client in healing process *see*
  responsibility for own health

Jesus Christ 133
jigsaw puzzle metaphor 80
Johnson, Don Hanlon 55, 176n
judgment 133, 135
  see also non-judgmental attitudes

Kahlbaum, Karl Ludwig 43
Kaptchuk, Ted 52, 53, 75, 90, 177n
Karrasch, Noah 31, 47, 55, 67, 89, 97,
    133, 139, 147, 157
  *Freeing Emotions and Energy Through
    Myofascial Release* 16, 114, 173n,
    179n
  Meet Your Body 19, 173n
  see also groin–gut–heart–head model
Keen, Lael Katharine 65
Kline, Maggie 34
Krippner, Stanley 86, 178n
Kübler-Ross, Elizabeth 87, 178n

layering model, bodywork 92–3
Leonard-Segal, Andrea 37–8, 174n
Levine, Peter 87, 94, 151, 152, 166,
    175n, 177n
  and caring 67, 71, 73
  and healing models 58, 59
  publications
    Trauma-proofing Your Kids 34, 174n
    In an Unspoken Voice 33, 174n, 176n,
      178n, 179n
    Waking the Tiger 41, 60, 174n
  and reasons for ill-health 40, 42, 43
  on "Somatic Experiencing" 118
  and survival 118, 119
life choices 15–16
life-or-death power 22
listening 77, 79, 81
"little me" 125
Littlejohn, Carmen 89, 90, 178n

logic 49
Lowen, Alexander 57, 58
Lupton, Deborah 16, 173n

magician (healer category) 63, 64, 65,
    112, 117, 131
Mann, John 62
Man's Search for Meaning (Frankl) 44, 175n
May, Rollo 68, 177n
medical models 139
medical schools 68
*Medicine as Culture: Illness, Disease and the
  Body* (Lupton) 16, 173n
Meet Your Body (Karrasch) 16, 173n
Mills, Stacey 68, 69
mirrors, healing 21, 26, 28, 73, 102
money 124
Moore, Thomas 50, 62, 82, 84, 97, 110,
    139, 176n
  Care of the Soul in Medicine 22, 148,
    173n, 175n, 178n, 179n, 180n
  on caring 70, 74–5
  on practitioner's need to be healed 100,
    102
motion starvation 61, 92
motives of healer/practitioner, questioning
    27, 98–9, 128
motor fibers 38–9
movement therapy 55, 60
Multi-Orgasmic Man, The (Chia and
  Abrams) 62, 126, 176n, 179n
music 28, 74
Mystery of Pain, The (Nelson) 51, 175n,
    178n

*Narrative Medicine: Honoring the Stories of
  Illness* (Charron) 80
Nelson, Douglas 51, 84–5, 175n, 178n
New Earth: Awakening to Your Soul's Purpose
  (Tolle) 41
nocebo effect 52
non-judgmental attitudes 69, 72–3, 77,
    94, 159
"non-profit" medical centers 27
Norris, Patricia 84, 178n
Northrup, Christiane 42
"noxious" people 95

nurturer (healer category) 63, 64, 65, 112, 117, 131
nutritional therapy 55, 56, 61, 64

observer, as participant 50–1
"one-size-fits-all" model, limitations 47, 56
open groin practitioner 113, 119, 120, 130–1, 165
open gut practitioner 113, 119, 120, 133, 134, 135, 167
open head practitioner 113, 119, 120, 132, 142, 149, 151, 171
open heart practitioner 113, 119, 120, 140, 142, 143, 169
openness/opening 34, 35, 112, 149, 150, 160
  opening one's heart 142, 164
orgasmic/orgone energy 57, 61, 124, 126, 127, 141, 151
Oriental medicine 56, 57, 127
Orlinsky, D. 35, 36, 174n
orthopedic surgery 55
Oschman, James 48, 53, 175n

pain 16, 40, 51, 58, 78, 83, 85, 88, 105, 106, 140, 143
  and caring 70, 72
  emotional/psychological 26, 41, 91, 109
  and feelings of safety 20, 23, 24, 25, 28
  release/resolve dilemma 93, 94, 95
  working with 99–100
Pain Free (Egoscue) 61
pain-body 41
"paint-by-number" therapist 17, 47
Painter, Jack 102–3, 104
  Deep Bodywork and Personal Development 22–3, 58, 173n, 176n, 179n
Pallardy, Pierre 138, 180n
parasympathetic nerve tone 33
participation of patron/client in therapy 28, 35, 42, 55
  cooperation 83–7
  see also responsibility for own health
Pathwork of Self Transformation, The (Pierrakos) 57

patron, definition 21, 22
pelvic floor 141
People of the Lie (Scott Peck) 42, 69, 101, 133, 175n, 177n, 179n, 180n
perfectionism 25–6, 58, 154
Persuasion and Healing (Jerome and Julia Frank) 35, 36, 66, 67
Pierrakos, Eva 57, 176n
Pierrakos, John 57, 58, 64, 90, 152, 176n
Pilates 60
placebo treatment 51–2, 53
"play dead" response see freeze response
Porges, Stephen 19, 34, 38, 40, 42, 67, 87, 91, 133, 152, 173n, 174n
positive group reality 116
post-traumatic stress disorder (PTSD) 40, 58, 141
practitioner centers, open and closed 165–72
  closed groin practitioner 113, 119, 120, 125, 131–2, 166
  closed gut practitioner 113, 119, 120, 136, 168
  closed head practitioner 113, 119, 120, 153–4, 172
  closed heart practitioner 113, 119, 120, 170
  open groin practitioner 113, 119, 120, 130–1, 165
  open gut practitioner 113, 119, 120, 133, 134, 135, 167
  open head practitioner 113, 119, 120, 132, 142, 149, 151, 171
  open heart practitioner 113, 119, 120, 140, 142, 143, 169
presence 117
processes (of practitioner), appropriate disclosures concerning 104–6
profit maximization, health providers 20, 27–8
prolonging of life, unnecessary 20
psychopathic personality 64
psychosomatic problems 25, 32, 58, 60, 109
  see also emotional blockages; pain
psychotherapy 56, 60
PTSD (post-traumatic stress disorder) 40, 58, 141

purpose for living 44
purpose safety 139–45

quality of life 20

reductionist thinking 48–9
reflective listening 81
Reich, Wilhelm 57, 58, 61, 90, 127, 152
reiki healing 55, 61
relationship difficulties 109–10
relaxation 38
Remen, Rachel Naomi 42, 77–8, 175n, 177n
re-moral-izing of clients 36, 37, 44, 67
  see also demoralization
repression 42, 58
rescuer (healer category) 63, 64, 65, 112, 117, 131
resilience 15, 19, 23, 26, 83, 99, 116
  fascial 59
  non-resilience 44
  and reasons for ill-health 34, 37, 38, 40
respiratory disorders 141
responsibility for own health 15, 19, 20, 23, 35, 69, 83, 160
  see also participation of patron/client in therapy
Revolutionary Trauma Release Process, The (Berceli) 23, 174n
Road Less Travelled, The (Scott Peck) 128, 179n
Roberts, R. 28, 173n
Rolf, Ida/Rolfing 59, 60, 72, 90, 93, 150
Rolf Institute, Boulder (Colorado) 47
root/survival (first) chakra 114, 115, 127, 158
round-earth theory 47
running 40
safety
  clarity 147–55
  creating 39–40, 75–8, 159
  demonstrating 15
  feeling safe 15, 19–29, 37
  feeling unsafe 19, 23, 24, 37, 40, 42, 76
  intuitive versus scientific 49
  practitioners' concepts of 76

purpose 139–45
satisfaction 123–32
self-esteem 133–8
sage (healer category) 63, 64, 65, 112, 117, 131
Sarno, John 25, 37–8, 42, 49, 60, 80, 82, 174n, 177n
satisfaction safety 123–32
Schedlowski, Manfred 52
Schulz, Mona Lisa 42, 123, 136–7, 140, 149
  All is Well 25, 49, 114–15, 173n, 174n, 175n, 179n, 180n
Schutz, Will 36–7, 95, 174n, 178n
Schwartz, Jack 79, 84, 177n
Schweitzer, Albert 49
science
  evidence-based medicine 47, 49, 50, 52, 148
  and facts 48, 49
  information overload 49, 133
  versus intuition 17, 47–53, 161
  reductionist thinking 48–9
  and stories 48, 49, 53
Scott Peck, M. 42, 69, 140
  People of the Lie 101, 133, 175n, 177n, 179n, 180n
  Road Less Travelled 128, 179n
self, working on 100, 105
self-awareness 15, 26, 112–13
self-determination 102
self-disclosure, appropriate level 104–6
self-esteem 42
  lack of 36–7, 137
  safety 133–8
self-help 15
self-image 24
selfishness 35
self-judgment 133
self-relatedness 35, 36
self-respect 23, 31, 35
serotonin 39
settings, care work 75–7
sexual energy 57, 123, 127, 128, 132, 168
  flow/movement 61, 125, 126
  stuck 126, 131

sexual/sacral (second) chakra 114, 115, 127
blocks 123–4
shallow breathing 32–3, 34
"sham" treatment 51–2
shame 124–5
Shield, Benjamin 24, 173n, 175n, 176n, 177n, 178n
SHIP (Spontaneous Healing Intrapersonal Process) (Steenkamp) 41, 59, 174n
Short, Larry 62
shutting down 44
Smith, Stretton 14–15
solar plexus (third) chakra 114
solitude 100
"Somatic Experiencing" (Levine) 118
spinal cord 39
Spiritual Aspects of the Healing Arts (Chernin) 79
Spiritual Emergency: When Personal Transformation Becomes a Crisis (Grof) 70, 177n
spirituality/spiritual healing 47, 61, 62
Steenkamp, Jo 42, 59–60, 90, 102, 105, 152, 157, 177n, 178n, 179n, 181n
SHIP (Spontaneous Healing Intrapersonal Process) 41, 59, 174n
Still, Andrew Taylor 59
stress 34–5
anti-stress mechanism 38
stubbornness 154
stuck energy, releasing 69, 89, 92, 99, 131, 151
groin–gut–heart–head model 110, 111
healing models 56, 59, 61
sexual energy 126, 131
see also energy; trauma
surface knowledge, limitations of 101
survival 38, 109–21
Sykes Wylie, Mary 65–6, 176n
"sympath" 69, 93, 140, 145
sympathetic nerve tone 33
sympathy, versus empathy 68–9, 96

Tai Chi 61
Taylor, Kylea 47, 63, 84, 123, 129, 131, 138, 175n, 178n, 179n, 180n

Teaching with Love and Logic (Fay and Funk) 86, 178n
Tension Myositis Syndrome (TMS) 25–6, 37–8, 41, 49, 58, 60
tests, unnecessary 20
therapeutic relationships 21–2, 26–7, 51
therapy visits, use of 91
third eye (sixth) chakra 114
Thomas, Richard 94
three-layered being model (Pierrakos) 57
throat (fifth) chakra 114, 115, 150
time 116–17
Time Magazine 20
TMS (Tension Myositis Syndrome) 25–6, 37–8, 41, 49, 58, 60
Tolle, Eckhart 31, 41, 125, 139, 174n, 175n, 179n, 180n
touching 31, 40, 51, 89, 98, 138, 151, 159
healing models 59, 65
safety, creating 77, 78
sexual energy blockages 127, 128, 129, 130, 132
trauma
airplane crash of author 13, 14, 80–1
deep-rooted, refusing to feel 43–4
ego centers 111
feelings of 24, 60
and holding one's breath 23, 31, 32, 36, 44
old and stored 14, 20, 92
post-traumatic stress disorder (PTSD) 40, 58, 141
releasing/resolving 34, 41, 43, 74, 161
communication skills 78–9, 83
healing models 58–9, 59, 60
needs of practitioner 103
release/resolve dilemma 89–96, 136
see also stuck energy, releasing
versus stress and anxiety 34–5
Trauma Informed Care 34
Trauma Release Process 41, 58–9
Trauma-proofing Your Kids (Levine and Kline) 34, 174n
Twerski, A.J. 37, 174n
Twilight Zone (television) 94, 144

uncertainty principle (Heisenberg) 50
underlying issues, resolving 89
unfinished business 25, 32, 111
United States, Unity church movement 14
Unity church movement, United States 14
unknown, fear of facing 26
Upledger, John 24, 118

vagus nerve 33, 38, 40, 57, 133, 141
validation, external/internal 20, 69, 73,
    106
    lack of 111
visceral manipulation 61

Waking the Tiger (Levine) 41, 60, 174n
Watts, Alan 148
Wisdom of Insecurity, The (Watts) 148
woundedness 24, 26
    wounded healer 99, 102

Yoga 61
You Can Heal Your Life (Hay) 25

Zanier, E. 50, 175n

CPI Antony Rowe
Eastbourne, UK
June 20, 2023